The Book of
Raw Fruit and Vegetable
Juices and Drinks

The Book That Tells You:

- the common fruit that contains more vitamin C, bite for bite, than an orange.
- the vegetable that has more protein than a steak.
- the largest plant on earth without a woody stem.
- if diabetics have trouble obtaining vitamin A from vegetables.
- what natural juice can help the pain of gout.
- the natural juice formulas that can aid which specific illnesses.
- how you prepare syrup of black currant.
- if dandelions are good to eat.
- what natural means you should use to stay regular.

All of This and More . . . Yours for the Reading in

The Book of Raw Fruit and Vegetable Juices and Drinks

The Book of
Raw Fruit and Vegetable Juices and Drinks

William H. Lee, R.Ph., Ph.D.

Keats Publishing, Inc.   New Canaan, Connecticut

With grateful acknowledgement to the pioneers of natural therapy:

Dr. N.W. Walker	*Susan E. Charmine*	*Gayelord Hauser*
Dr. L. Newman	*Carlson Wade*	*Carlton Fredericks*
Dr. Jean Valnet	*Paavo Airola*	*Kurt W. Donsbach*

The information contained in this book is in no way to be considered as medical advice. It is advisable to seek professional advice or consult your physician in every case where you are in doubt about your health, or when you have continuing symptoms.

**The Book of
Raw Fruit and Vegetable Juices and Drinks**

Copyright © 1982 by William Lee, R.Ph., Ph.D.

ISBN: 0-87983-306-8

Library of Congress Catalog Number 82-82323

Printed in the United States of America

Keats Publishing, Inc.,
27 Pine Street, New Canaan, Connecticut 06840

to
my wife and my mother
with deepest love and
gratitude

CONTENTS

1. Plant Life—The Link between Life and Death   1
2. Enzymes—the Magic Molecules   4
3. Why Drink Raw Juice?   10
4. The Nutrients in Raw Juices   16
5. Juice Therapy   26
6. How to Buy a Juicer   70
7. What and Why Are Those Wonder Nutrients in Fruits and Vegetables?   76
8. Juice in Sickness and in Health   88
9. A Cleansing Fast (with Juices)   112
10. What's What in Food and on Labels   116
11. Juiced for Fun   129
12. Please Squeeze the Fruit   139
13. You Are Today What You Ate Yesterday   148
14. The Easiest Diet You Ever Tried   160
    Index   169

**The Book of
Raw Fruit and Vegetable
Juices and Drinks**

1. *Plant Life—the Link between Life and Death*

::

ALL ANIMAL LIFE—including man, since man and animal have a common life-style on this planet—is nourished directly or indirectly by plants.

Plant life is the processing device by which Nature extracts food elements from the sun, soil and water and prepares them for assimilation. And plants provide more than food; the only breathable oxygen produced by Nature is from the leaves of vegetation. So, in truth, human life is dependent upon the vegetable kingdom.

Ancient alchemists searched for a process that would transmute base metal into gold, and never found it. Yet plants do that mysterious task with ease. Inorganic, lifeless mineral matter is converted into living organic material which, when presented to the human body, is hungrily absorbed. These inorganic substances, if obtained without the intervention of plant life, cannot sustain life—in fact, many of them are poisonous and will destroy tissue. Take the case of oxalic acid, which is found in combination with sodium, potassium, calcium, iron and manganese in the juice of many plants. When oxalic acid is prepared by man by oxidizing sugar and starch with nitric acid, it is one of the most powerful poisons known. One dram will quickly prove fatal, destroying the organic structure of any tissue it touches, eating away the tissues of the mouth, stomach, duodenum, finally perforating the peritoneum and, approximately thirty minutes after ingestion, bringing death after great pain and suffering.

Yet the same acid in the form of iron oxalate, potassium or sodium or calcium oxalates as found in rhubarb, sorrel leaves, cinchona, oak bark, spinach, etc., is quite harmless and is consumed by man and animals in large quantities.

Another example is inorganic sulfur. The injurious effects of this mineral result from its affinity for iron, for its destruction of enzymes and ferments, and from the generation of acids within the organism. It steals iron from the blood and from food in the stomach, forming iron sulphide which constipates the digestive tract. It robs nascent hydrogen from fluids and tissues, forming a foul-smelling gas. It is the smell of rotten eggs and decaying matter.

On the other hand, the organic sulfur in onions, watercress and garlic is healthful, virtuous and non-poisonous. They are delightful foods and condiments, adding much to salads and other meals. In fact, the juices of garlic and onion are helpful in medicine and are being used to regulate blood pressure.

The difference between inorganic and organic is no longer important once the material has been processed by man's greatest friends, the abundant plant life gracing this planet.

Scientists tell us that our bodies are composed of more than twenty mineral elements, all of which must be replenished from food sources, and all of which must be processed by plants before we can assimilate them—even the iron we get from liver, for example, was assimilated by the animal from plants.

So, too, all the other nutrients, including protein, vitamins, and enzymes, whether taken in from animal or plant foods, are originally derived from plants.

The best and most abundant sources of most of these minerals and nutrients are fruits and vegetables. But not, unhappily the fruits and vegetables most of us eat, the way we prepare them. Processing and cooking destroy nutritive values and often add harmful elements, ranging from the chemicals in processed food to aluminum from cooking pots.

It is fresh, raw fruits and vegetables that are the true source of the vital nutrients. The rub is that eating enough of them can be troublesome, time-consuming, and, for people with digestive or dental problems, painful or impossible.

Juicing the fruits and vegetables—reducing them to a flavorful, easily consumed liquid—is a way to boost the health benefits derived from them far beyond those that can be obtained from eating them. A daily intake of raw juices will guarantee that the body is receiving a good part of its quota of building material for its trillions of cells.

In the rest of this book I shall discuss the nature of the various juices, their use in therapy and for maintaining health, and the elements to be found in them.

Among the most remarkable of these elements are the enzymes—perhaps the most easily destroyed of all the vital nutrients—which are dealt with in the next chapter.

2. Enzymes, The Magic Molecules

WITHOUT ENZYMES, life would be impossible—the body would starve to death in the midst of plenty. Enzymes are necessary to convert food into energy and living cells. Vitamins can do their work only in the presence of enzymes. Enzymes are the catalysts which bring about the complicated chemical changes that prepare food for assimilation and digestion.

Salivary Enzymes: As soon as food is put into the mouth or, if the food looks or smells good, at the very prospect of eating it, several enzymes are released by the salivary glands to begin digestion even before the food enters the stomach. That's why the old advice of chewing each mouthful of food thirty times before swallowing is as valid today as it was when it was first stated. The enzyme ptyalin starts the preliminary work of digestion by combining with moisture to attack the carbohydrates in the food and reduce them to maltose, the predigested form of starch, or energy-producing sugar.

Stomach Enzymes: After being thoroughly chewed, the food is swallowed and enters the stomach, where the gastric juices contain new enzymes to continue the digestive process. The stomach has been signaled by the sight, the smell and the taste of food to start releasing the needed chemicals from the glands. That's one of the reasons for foods to be prepared in a manner that will appeal to the senses. Food that is appealing and is anticipated will be digested more thoroughly.

The enzyme rennin handles milk, causing it to coagulate and changing the milk protein (casein) into amino acids which the body can use. Rennin also works on the minerals of milk and cheese to make them available for assimilation into the system. The calcium, phosphorous, potassium, magnesium present in the foods can then be transported by the bloodstream to all the cells that need them—the bones, teeth, nerves, organs, etc.

The enzymes pepsin and lipase are also present in the stomach. Pepsin is the chief protein-splitter, breaking down long chains into shorter chains that the body can handle. Lipase works on fat and splits it into forms which the body uses for nourishment.

Hydrochloric acid presents a problem: is it to be considered an enzyme or even more than an enzyme? It breaks down protein foods and the tough fiber of vegetable cells to release the protein, minerals, vitamins, etc., but, because it's an acid it also destroys bacteria in the stomach, and is thus part of the defense system of the body. It also helps to regulate the acid-base balance in the system and, without adequate hydrochloric acid, there would be no way to liberate iron from food so it can be converted into a form the body can use. Hydrochloric acid, or rather the lack of it, can be one of the most important factors affecting digestion. A low level can cause excess gas, incomplete digestion, malnutrition and a host of other uncomfortable or debilitating symptoms. The hydrochloric acid level is the first thing to be checked when there is extreme upper or lower gas, burping after meals, flatulence and so on.

Intestinal enzymes: The next step for the food is into the small intestine where it is subjected to more enzymes to extract and transform the vital nutrients from the food into assimilable form. There's bile to emulsify fats, then pancreatic lipase to change the fat into fatty acids (they keep the skin and mucous membrane in good condition, help in building the linings of nerve and brain tissue and help in all healing processes). Then there's tripsin to continue the work begun by pepsin and rennin; and lactase, streapsin, amylopsin, and so on and on.

There are over 600 different types of enzymes, and each one of them performs a separate and vital function. Enzymes are present in every one of the billions of cells in your body. Without enzymes the body cannot convert food into energy or transform protein, carbohydrates, fats, vitamins and other nutrients into muscle, bone, hair, skin, organs, glands, hormones and so on. Without enzymes, wounds would not heal. Enzymes protect against inflammation, dissolve clots, erase scars, counteract the adverse effects of drugs, aid in the coagulation of blood, promote oxygenation of blood and are even involved in your sex life.

Enzymes are responsible for the normal healthy function of all of your bodily processes, for your mental and physical health. These miraculous molecules are the special youth-factors created by Nature and provided in plants. And they are most readily and easily obtained from natural foods in their raw state. When you eat raw foods, the body is supplied with all of the enzymes necessary for digestion and assimilation of the nutrients found in those foods. Enzymes are not stored; after they do their job they are destroyed, and the body has to obtain or manufacture new batches. That's why the quality of the food you eat is so important.

Enzyme destruction: The day man discovered how to cook was the day he opened Pandora's Box of disease, premature aging and death. Temperatures over 122°F. are lethal to enzymes, which means, when fruit and vegetables are cooked—all too often overcooked—all enzymes are destroyed.

Therefore, if you want the power of the enzyme undiminished, you have to eat your foods in their natural, raw state. This can be easy or it can be difficult. Part of it, the easy part, is tasting fruits, vegetables, nuts, seeds, honey, legumes, etc., just the way they are when they come from the ground, the tree or the hive. You'll find they are more delicious raw than cooked, and easier to digest than cooked food—provided you haven't totally destroyed your digestive system with devitalized food, overcooked, oversoftened, undernourishing.

If that's so, you have to give yourself time to rebuild your system so it can adjust to a new eating system. Start gradually by adding raw food and juices to your diet. As your system begins to enjoy the unexpected rush of good health, add more and more raw foods until your diet consists of about two-thirds raw and one-third cooked and processed food.

Primitive man living on raw fruits, nuts, berries or raw milk discovered an ancient method of preserving by fermentation. He used enzymes to make sour milk and sour cheese. He learned how to make bread rise with the help of enzymes. He lived with Nature and did not suffer from the diseases of civilization. Cooking destroys enzymes and other nutrients and detracts from our stomachs' innate ability to digest food. The enzymatic system can be wooed back into action by starting with juices. The raw juice-raw food-raw fruit-raw honey program discussed in this book will provide foods that practically digest themselves.

Modern farming methods are designed to make profits and not to deliver nutritious food. Fruits and vegetables are picked before they mature and sprayed with chemicals to look ripe. Canning procedures destroy enzymes and vitamins. The length of time between picking, packing, transportation, cold storage, packaging and the actual purchase by the consumer, depletes much of the nutrient value. Other practices which remove vitamins and add refined sugar contribute calories and destroy nutrition.

First aid for extra enzymes:

1. Eat as much of your food raw as you possibly can.
2. Eat foods as soon after they have been harvested as possible.
3. Eat foods as soon after you buy them as possible.
4. Store foods in a chiller. Cold does not destroy enzymes. Heat does!
5. In the winter use frozen raw fruits and vegetables but eat them immediately after thawing.
6. Don't cook vegetables; steam them and only long enough to make them chewable.
7. Chew, chew, chew your food. Enzyme action begins in the mouth. Don't train your body to cease its activity anywhere.
8. Make fermented foods at home, like sauerkraut, yogurt or kefir. They are enzyme-rich and pre-digested.
9. Use raw grains and sprouted seeds. Make your own Muesli for breakfast.
10. Buy a juice extractor for enzyme-loaded drinks. Drink juices before meals or with meals but never after meals (don't mix fruit juice with vegetable juice). They'll cause gas. Go on a juice fast for a day or two to let your stomach rest.
11. Take natural supplements and a good vitamin/mineral

tablet supplement. Some natural supplements are brewer's yeast, honey, papaya, and kelp.

3. *Why Drink Raw Juice?*

LONG LIFE should be our goal—so long as it is enjoyed, not endured. Abstinence from dangerous, highly processed, civilized foods is one of the foremost requirements for good health. There is a drastic need for unsprayed products from fertile farms, for the heat-labile nutrients which can only be obtained through adequate intake of raw foods. When the dangerous foods of civilized life are omitted from the diet, not only does health improve, but the fun in eating is restored.

Health or profit? Ask anyone what they'd choose and health has to win. But the food industry, with its multi-billion-dollar investment, must show a profit, and it's done at the expense of health—yours and mine.

Let's examine just a few of the products found on the market shelves. Start with the packaged cereals, frozen french fries, and ketchup—each of them with substantial amounts of refined sugar added to a basically wholesome food.

The value of sugar in nutrition is based entirely on its ability to supply energy fuel to the body. Foods rich in sugar are therefore of great importance, and, when in combination with other nutrients, provide the body with exceptional nutriment. The key word is "combination."

Mankind has always had a "sweet tooth" because it

was necessary for survival. Early man lived on fruits and vegetables and, when he was able, some small amounts of fish and meat. The mainstay of his existence, however, was the food that didn't want to eat him first! When fruit is mature it is at its sweetest, and when it is at its sweetest it also contains the most vitamins, minerals and enzymes. The caveman who let himself be guided by his nose and his "sweet tooth" chose the ripest, most mature fruit. He obtained all of his nutritional requirements, remained healthy, and barring unforseen accidents, had healthy children. The caveman who ate unripe fruits did not get a full complement of nutrients and probably passed less healthy genes along. In those days only the healthiest children and adults survived (and we may be getting back to those days, like it or not).

As time passed, the chief sources of sugar were honey, ripe fruit and sugar cane and, lately, the sugar beet. That's when the real trouble started. Mechanical methods were developed to separate the sugar from the remainder of the plant. In the beginning, the end product was brown sugar. It had a nice taste and still contained some of the vitamins and minerals originally present in the plant. Progress continued until the modern processor was able to carry the sugar cane or other sugar source into a complete state of refinement. The product was pure white in color and the last traces of vitamins and minerals were now gone. That is the refined sugar most of us have on our table. That is the sugar we find in our cereals, bread, cookies, in our ketchup, on our french fried potatoes, and in a host of other foods. It is an unbalanced food, devoid of all minerals, vitamins and other accessory nutrients. If our cave ancestors had had the advantages of refined sugar, we wouldn't be here now!

When this product is put into our bodies, the body must use up vitamins and other elements to try to digest it and utilize it as quickly as it can. The individual cannot handle refined sugar in the 99 percent pure state; our bodies were not designed to cope with it. What usually happens is an overreaction that burns up the sugar very rapidly, necessitating more sugar intake to keep the blood-sugar level near normal. If this intake continues for any length of time the organs involved wear down and artificial means of sugar control must be instituted.

Does this mean we have to live sugar-free? Not at all. The problem is not sugar, only refined sugar. The natural sweetness available in fruit juices can satisfy the sweetest tooth, and the sweetness is combined with all of the natural nutrients necessary for its digestion.

Now move to the canned-vegetable aisle. The rise of the frozen food industry has reduced the consumption of fresh fruits and vegetables but has done little to affect the consumption of canned products. This has serious consequences in terms of health. Canning must include heat-processing. Most vegetables are blanched before canning, which causes some loss of nutritional factors. Then, during the canning process itself, they are cooked for 24 to 40 minutes at a temperature of 240° F. or higher to achieve complete sterilization. Without sterilization the food would spoil.

There is no way for food that is sterilized to retain its nutrition. Enzymes in particular are completely destroyed, while much of the vitamin content is seriously depleted. In addition, many canned products are heavily salted, and, in the case of commercial fruit juices and fruits, sugar may be added as a sweetening agent. Artificial flavor and color may also be added as well as preservatives. When that is added to the possibility of month after month on a shelf, the product is thoroughly devitalized and incapable of meeting basic nutritional standards.

However, the food industry is not the only villain. There is also "murder in the kitchen"—what the average cook can do to reduce fresh vegetables into a nutritionless mess is really mass murder.

The first thing that is done is to remove the peel— and there goes a batch of minerals. Then it is dropped into water and heated without mercy. Say "so long" to the water-soluble vitamins B-complex and C. The heat destroys the enzymes and the minerals are left behind in the water. The sink gets more vitamins and minerals than you do. It's not done with malice. Usually a cook learns from a parent, who learned from a parent, who learned from someone who knew nothing about nutrition or a balanced diet. In some cases it didn't matter, because times were hard and anything was better than an empty stomach. However, times are different and healthful eating is many times cheaper than unhealthful eating. It is knowledge that's important.

Why did we start to cook things in the first place? It must have begun when we adopted the practice of eating meat. The human stomach is not acidic enough to digest meat in chunk form. A cat has many more times the amount of acid in its stomach than a human does. A cat can eat a mouse whole and be able to digest it down to the tip of its tail. Our stomachs are more suited to digest fruits, vegetables and grains. What we really do when we cook meat is to partially digest it with fire.

That still doesn't explain why we started to cook vegetables. The answer is that some vegetables are too hard to chew and are softened in hot water. It's true that the cells of plants are composed of cellulose, a rather firm material, and it is also true that the nutrients are locked up in those cells and the cell wall must be broken down in order to liberate the nutritional material so our stomachs can take advantage of the treasures Nature has prepared. But cooking in water removes most of the nutritional content. Steaming for a few minutes is much better, but mechanical juicing is far better still.

The juicer splits the food without heat, squeezes out the nutrient-bearing juice and leaves only the pulp behind. All the vitamins, minerals, enzymes, co-enzymes, sugars and trace minerals go into your glass. And it's all natural.

On December 5, 1981 the *New York Times* featured an article about the risks of lung cancer and the reduction of the risk with the use of beta-carotene. Beta-carotene is a precursor of vitamin A; that is, the body can convert beta-carotene into vitamin A. There are two main sources of vitamins: one is the plant kingdom and the other is the animal kingdom. There is, of course, the chemical laboratory, but I'm thinking of natural sources at the moment. Fish-liver oil supplies Vitamin A as do eggs, cheese, and milk, while the beta-carotene form is found in carrots, squash, dandelion greens, cantaloupe, and most yellow-orange fruits and vegetables.

The article was concerned with a nineteen-year study of cigarette smoking and lung cancer and involved a group of almost 2,000 men. The study began in 1957 and when the data was analyzed, a link was found between dietary beta-carotene and a lowered incidence of cancer. The study did not determine whether it was vitamin A or the beta-carotene that reduced the risk, and a further study was conducted at a number of universities. The answer was that the protection came from the plant source, beta-carotene.

The article goes on to explore carotene's apparent potential for resisting cancer and its aid in the restoration of body tissue as well as its role in protecting vision.

The point is that Nature has an abundance of protective material that is needed by the body, and we just have to find a way to get it. People with any kind of mouth problem—and there are millions of them ranging from lost teeth, to poor bone structure, to ill-fitting dentures—find it difficult to chew the number of carrots needed for a day's supply of beta-carotene. A juicer will take five carrots, smash the pulp and give a glass of healthful, golden juice in less than five minutes! And who said we have to stop there? Later in this book we'll see many different vegetable and fruit sources of vitamins and other nutrients that can even be used to assist the body in recovering from certain illnesses.

4. *The Nutrients in Raw Juices*

THE AMOUNT of nutrients you get from any glass of raw juice depends on the protein, sugar, vitamins, minerals, and enzymes in the original food which you juiced. It also depends on how much you drink and how quickly you drink it after it has been juiced. Most of the value is retained if you drink it at once. The longer it stands, the greater the chance of the vital components being lost. So make enough juice for yourself or your family and make it fresh each time.

What approximately is in your carrot juice and how much? Most food composition tables don't list raw juices, so there's no easy source of information. If you use half a pound of carrots, you will find that your glass of juice contains:

Vitamin C	15 mg	Iron	1.3 mg
Niacin	1.1 mg	Phosphorus	67 mg
Vitamin B2	.1 mg	Calcium	69 mg
Vitamin B1	.1 mg	Carbohydrate	18 grams
Vitamin A	20,460 I.U.	Protein	2 grams
Potassium	635 mg	Calories	78
Sodium	88 mg		

The amount of beta-carotene (vitamin A) and the amount of phosphorus you get from that juice is enormous. These are both essential to health. The potassium is especially important if you, like most people, use a lot of salt. Potassium helps to balance this unwise use.

The following chart shows the amount of nutrients you can expect from one pound of fruit. Wash the fruit carefully with soap and water and rinse. Take the left-over pulp and save it; it's the fiber, and very important to help keep the process of elimination functioning. Use it in soup. Add some yogurt, chicken stock and onions. If it is sweet fruit, turn it into a dessert with chopped nuts and shredded coconut. Be inventive.

We'll cover the rest of the fruits when we go over their individual therapeutic uses. This was just to give you an idea of the range of nutrients we take for granted and the amount of nutrients we throw away without being aware of it. If the amounts seem small when compared to the amounts shown on the label of your vitamin bottle, don't worry. These are natural components and every bit is available to the body. It's not that I am against taking supplemental vitamins; I'm not. In fact, I believe in using supplements along with natural vitamin sources. One reinforces the other. I *am* against using supplemental vitamins and eating junk foods. Nutrition must come from food and supplements in order to be effective. Taking vitamin tablets and eating junk food is like taking out a burglary insurance policy and leaving your front door open. Sooner or later your policy will be cancelled.

It's easier to buy orange juice in a container? It's cheaper than buying a juicer? That's the most expensive savings you ever thought of. Let's examine the Food and Drug Administration proposals on certain orange juice products. There are nine pages and here are some of the products discussed:

1. Water extracted soluble orange products

NUTRIENTS IN ONE POUND OF FRUIT

Fruit	Calcium	Phos.	Iron	Sodium	Vit. A	B1	B2	Niacin	C	Potassium
Apricots	72	98	2.1	4	11,510	.14	.16	2.6	42	733
Blackberries	138	82	3.9	4	860	.14	1.18	1.6	90	1,198
Blueberries	63	54	4.2	4	420	.13	.25	1.9	58	338
Cherries	92	79	1.7	8	4,170	.21	.25	1.7	42	797
Cranberries	61	44	2.2	9	190	.13	.09	.4	47	357
Grapefruit	36	36	.9	2	300	.08	.04	.4	84	300
Grapes, white	48	81	1.6	12	400	.21	.11	1	18	698
Honeydew	40	46	1.1	34	120	.13	.09	1.8	65	717
Oranges	136	66	1.3	3	660	.33	.13	1.3	166	662

2. Dehydrated water extracted soluble orange solids
3. Pulverized oranges
4. Dehydrated, pulverized oranges
5. Dehydrated extract of pulverized oranges
6. Orange pulp for manufacturing
7. Dehydrated orange pulp for manufacturing
8. Noncarbonated orange flavored beverage
9. Concentrate for flavored beverage
10. Orange drinks and diluted orange juice
11. Powdered flavored beverage
12. Concentrate for diluted orange juice beverages
13. Orange juice drink and blended orange juice drink

The list goes on and on, and after each designation appears a lengthy description of how much orange has to be in the drink, what chemical additives are and are not permitted, whether vitamin C shall be declared as "vitamin C added" or "with added vitamin C".

They permit anti-caking agents, foaming agents, browning inhibiters, acidifiers, clouding agents, stabilizers, thickeners, buffers, artificial colors and synthetic vitamins. . . .

Do you still want to buy a carton of orange juice? Plus, even if it's 100 percent pure, it's been pasteurized! The heat required for pasteurization is enough to drive off or devitalize most of the vitamin C. If you want orange water buy a commercial juice; if you want orange juice, juice it yourself.

I really shouldn't condemn all commercial products. There is a quick frozen, 100 percent real orange juice that is in the freezer at the local supermarket. It's a concentrate and contains almost all of the nutrients present in fresh oranges. So I'll back off a bit as far as the frozen concentrate is concerned but not a bit on the orange drinks.

What I have said about fruits goes double for vegetables. They are wonderful sources of nutritional elements. We've taken a look at a pound of carrots and now we'll examine a few others.

When the early caveman left his home in the morning, hungry and thirsty, he ate whatever was at hand. Leaves, fruits, berries, roots, tubers and anything else. He wasn't fastidious. Maybe he shook the carrot once or twice to get rid of the dirt and maybe he didn't. The dirt, clinging to the roothairs, contained needed minerals. The carrots and the fruits contained most of the other nutrients and the grains supplied the needed protein. We, of course, must wash our vegetables very carefully to get rid of any clinging pesticide. Use the skins when you can, but avoid skins that may have been dyed like oranges, apples or red potatoes.

One pound of any of the following will supply (mg):

	Beets	Beet Greens*	Broccoli	Cabbage	Parsley
Calcium	51	302	364	200	921
Phosphorus	105	102	276	118	286
Iron	2.2	8.4	3.9	1.6	28.1
Sodium	190	330	53	82	204
Potassium	1064	1448	1352	951	3298
Vit. A	80	15490	8840	530	38560
Vit. B1	.1	.24	.35	.22	.54
Vit. B2	.15	.55	.81	.2	1.19
Niacin	1.2	1	3.2	1.3	5.6
Vit. C	32	76	400	192	780

*Look at all of the good nutrition you've been throwing away

I'm not happy about putting list after list of items to prove a point. It gets boring after a while, and once you have been convinced of a fact it does little good to keep

there's no power on earth that will make it grow. What most people do is feed dead food to live cells and then expect peak performance. The body will respond for a long time by robbing the needed elements from various parts of itself, but inevitably degeneration must set in unless new supplies are obtained.

We are the only inhabitants of this planet that haven't learned how to feed ourselves, but we're trying. If you have a cat or a dog, you know what they do if they get sick. They nose around, sniffing several grasses and when they find the one they need, they eat it. They trust their instinct and they get well. We use our intelligence when we should use intelligence plus instinct plus knowledge, because our food intelligence has been perverted by many factors.

Far too few people realize the value of fresh, raw vegetables and fruits in their diet. Eating raw food occasionally doesn't help a great deal. The body cannot store a number of vitamins and minerals, and needs a daily supply. One of the greatest discoveries in the field of nutrition was that Nature never delivers isolated vitamins and minerals—she always gives them to us in combinations. We have isolated many of these, but there are many still remaining to be discovered. Many people cannot eat a raw salad. I've given some reasons, but there are others:

They don't like salads.

They have artificial dentures and can't chew raw vegetables.

They haven't time to chew. They have to get back to work!

Their stomachs are sensitive to raw food.

They can't digest raw vegetables.

I can't argue with them because they may be right! In any of the cases above, perhaps only 1 percent of the raw vegetables will be assimilated due to poor chewing ability or digestive lack. The answer is . . . juice.

There's an old adage in advertising: when writing an ad you must tell them in the headline; then you must tell them why you told them; then tell them again. I believe a juicer belongs in every home and I'm telling you again:

1. Persons with chewing difficulties can take their raw food in the form of juice.

2. A person who has no time can get all of the nourishment of a salad in the form of juice. It is quickly and easily consumed.

3. Most people with stomach troubles cannot eat raw foods, yet carrot juice is soothing, healing and nourishing. There is no roughage to irritate stomach lining or ulcers.

4. Only the cellulose is discarded when a vegetable is made into juice. The vitamins, minerals and other nutrients can revitalize the body with the least amount of effort by the body.

5. If a person is sickly, with a poor appetite, juices will provide nutrients without having to force food into an unwilling stomach.

6. While most of what I've said is directed at mature individuals, I do not mean to restrict the use of juices to them alone. Little babies will love carrot juice mixed with milk, and it won't curdle. If they won't eat vegetables, let them have the benefits of carrot juice. Adolescents frequently have poor eating habits and sometimes a lack of certain vitamins and minerals contribute to a pimply face. Juices can help

provide the missing nutrients and help to clear up diet-caused acne.
7. Above all else, raw vegetable juice taken daily insures the body its daily quota of building material. Most people drag themselves through life not supplying their body with enough fuel to keep it running easily. They could, if they wanted, enjoy much more of the trip.

There is in every one of us an amazing store of untapped knowledge that we tend to put aside in favor of schooling. But all of that schooling cannot put together one single cell and make it live. Nature puts together five hundred billion cells, each in its proper place and each doing its special job and, in nine months' time, produces a baby.

By following Nature's laws, consuming only what the body needs and allowing the body to direct its healing, we can correct many problems and enjoy every day.

5. Juice Therapy

RAW JUICE therapy does not conflict with other forms of treatment and is frequently used in conjunction with standard methods. Avoid self-diagnosis of a complaint, especially if it is serious. No practitioner would diagnose his own complaint without seeking a second opinion, yet many laymen do just that. They may be right many times, but mistakes can happen; so, when there is a serious complaint, do not treat yourself but do seek out a physician sympathetic to natural therapies.

The materials about natural sources are arranged alphabetically to make references as easy as possible. I have not separated fruits from vegetables because, again, it's easy this way. I've included the botanical origin as well as the common name in case one or more vegetables share a name and it's important to know which is which.

Some juices are very strong and you need to use just a little. Others are less powerful in their effect and can be taken a pint at a time. Dosage will be indicated for all juices. Most therapeutic formulas are combinations of juices. This also will be indicated. Pure juice can be assimilated in from ten to fifteen minutes compared to hours required for the assimilation of a complete fruit or vegetable. Put a juicer in your office and have a juice break instead of a coffee break. You'll feel and work better and that's the object of this book.

ALFALFA

Botanical Origin: *Medicago sativa*
Common Name: *Lucerne, Buffalo Herb*

Alfalfa is one of the oldest cultivated plants. The Arabs, who called it "Father of all foods," used it as a feed for their magnificent horses. When they noticed that the animals were able to run faster and were stronger than other horses, they began to eat it themselves with beneficial results.

The benefits are partially due to alfalfa's extraordinarily long roots. They extend deep into the earth—some as far as forty feet or more—down into the subsoil to extract the minerals shallow-rooted plants can't reach. Normally only trees could tap these nutrients.

Alfalfa contains vitamins A,B,D,E,K and U. It is one of the two known land plants that contain vitamin B12 (comfrey is the other one). It is also rich in vitamin C and calcium, iron, potassium, sodium, silicon, magnesium and trace elements. Alfalfa is also a source of eight different enzymes.

The chlorophyll molecule is designed much like our hemoglobin molecule. The basic difference is that plant blood is based on magnesium while human blood is based on iron. The elements around the core are remarkably similar. Interestingly enough, chlorophyll turns red under ultra-violet light while human blood turns green, the color of chlorophyll, under the same light. We find this to be one of the secrets of juice therapy.

Alfalfa is one of the richest chlorophyll foods we have. While the juice is too strong to take alone, it can be combined with carrot juice and the beneficial effects of both are increased. It can benefit blood and heart conditions not caused by organic disturbance, be useful in the treatment of respiratory ills, help clear congested sinuses and, when combined with lettuce juice (drink a pint of the combination daily), has been reported to stimulate hair growth.

The protein content is similar to that of beef but not nearly as tasty. The leaves of the plant are rich in magnesium and can be made into a tea.

APPLE

Botanical Origin: *Pyrus Malus*
Common name: *Eve's Apple*

Some apples are an important source of vitamin C although oranges and lemons and tomatoes have a higher vitamin content. Apples also contain a lot of minerals, as well as pectin, malic acid and tannic acid, which are wonderful aids in purifying the intestinal area.

Apple juice is a blood purifier and general tonic and is helpful to the skin. It contains, in addition to vitamin C, vitamins B1, B2, niacin, carotene, vitamin B6, biotin and folic acid. There is also a lot of potassium and phosphorus. It's good for flushing the kidneys and controlling digestive upsets.

Apple juice should be made fresh and not stored even in the refrigerator, since it oxidizes quickly. Make it and drink it at once. Apple cider vinegar retains much of the health-giving qualities of the apple. Always buy vinegar that states it was made from the whole apple.

APRICOT

Botanical Origin: *Prunus armeniaca, Armeniaca vulgaris rosacea*

The name Apricot derives from the Latin *praecoquum,* "early ripening," because it ripens before its cousin, the peach. It is suspected that the golden apples of the Bible were really apricots, since the apples growing in that region at that time were of the crabapple type and of very poor quality.

The apricot contains just as much vitamin C whether it is gathered hard or ripened but the pro-vitamin A (beta-carotene) is greatest when the fruit has been allowed to tree-ripen. There is more than 200 percent more carotene in the ripe fruit.

Apricots contain:

vitamins A, B, C
beta-carotene
protein
lipids
trace elements including magnesium, phosphorus, iron, calcium, potassium, sodium, sulfur, manganese, cobalt and bromine.

Its main therapeutic use is in providing beta-carotene and also as a flavoring. Crack the apricot kernel open sometimes and grind the nut inside to add to the juice. It is one of the new sources of nitrilosides. The flavor is similar to almonds but slightly more bitter.

ASPARAGUS

Botanical Origin: *Asparagus officinalis*
Common Name: *Sparrow Grass*

Asparagus is a cousin of the orchid and a member of the lily family. In the United States we eat only the spears, but in other parts of the world the seeds are used as a coffee substitute and the berries are fermented into a drinkable liquid. In the Orient, the spears are candied with sugar and honey.

Long before it began to be eaten as a vegetable, asparagus had a reputation as a medicinal agent. It contains rutin, a bioflavonoid that contributes to the health of the tiny capillaries and an alkaloid, aspargine, which stimulates the kidneys, causing a strong diuretic effect. If asparagus is cooked, the amount of the alkaloid is reduced by a great deal; so if a diuretic effect is desired, use just a small amount of the juice.

Asparagus also contains a good amount of vitamin C, vitamin A and the B-complex group, as well as the minerals potassium, manganese and iron. Asparagus therapy will yield a strong color and odor to the urine, so don't let this surprise you or deter you from its use.

Botanically, asparagus is unusual in that there are male and female plants. The female may be recognized by both flower and seed pods, but both sexes are therapeutically active. The plant's growth is unusual since an individual spear may grow as much as ten inches in a single day.

AVOCADO

> **Botanical Origin:** *Persea americana, Persea gratissima*
> **Common Name:** *Alligator Pear*

The avocado is no relation to the pear, despite the name. It may have come about because of its shape which can be somewhat like a fat pear (although it is just as often round) or because its skin is rough like an alligator (although it is frequently smooth).

Avocados are native Americans originally grown in Mexico and Central America. They are extremely high in protein and much more like a nut than a fruit. The avocado contains a large supply of beta-carotene (three times as much in a ripe fruit as in an unripe fruit), and nutritionists have found eleven vitamins and seventeen minerals, making it a comprehensive storehouse of nutrition. There is a high level of oil which contains vitamins A, D and E and, although the calorie count is high, it is a very worthwhile food.

The juice is a good way of obtaining a balanced oil of avocado. It is an excellent penetrating oil when applied to the skin as an emollient and has no known sensitizing effects. It is ideal for soothing sensitive skin.

BANANA

> **Botanical Origin:** *Musa sapientum, Musa parasidiaca musaceae*
> **Common Name:** *Paradise Tree*

The banana is not grown on a tree nor is it a tree. It

is the largest plant on earth without a woody stem. It ranks very high on the nutritional table. It is richer in minerals than any other soft fruit except the mighty strawberry. Although it is high in calories, it can be used in reducing diets. It is a natural laxative, a soothing treat for ulcer or colitis sufferers, an aid in the treatment of ailments of the kidney. It is more healthful than potatoes and more digestible than meat.

The banana contains vitamins A, B-complex, C and E. It is very useful in supporting the energy level of elderly individuals if it is ripe. Green or underripe bananas have a heavy starch content that is difficult to digest, but that changes to digestible fruit sugar as the banana ripens.

BEANS (Green)

Botanical Origin: *Phaseolus vulgaris, Legume (papilionacrae)*

One of the advantages of using a juicer is that you don't throw any part of the food away. If you have the right kind of home juicer, everything is used—the stem, the seed, the peel, and the leaves if they are still intact.

Green beans contain a number of constituents that are valuable. Vitamins A, B-complex, C, chlorophyll, carbohydrates, and minerals including phosphorus, calcium, copper and cobalt.

It also is a rare source of one of the B-complex vitamins called inositol which is found mostly in the "strings."

Half a glass daily may be useful for rheumatism and gout, decreased urinary output and fatigue caused by overwork. It is also said to promote the normal action of the liver and the pancreas.

BEET (Red)

Botanical Origin: *Beta rubra, Beta vulgaris rapa*

The beet we eat is technically a beetroot and a relative of the sugar beet and chard. In ancient times only the leaves were eaten. The root was used as a medicine and as a snuff to promote sneezing (the white beet was best for that).

According to the Doctrine of Signatures, which suggests that every plant illustrates its medical purpose either by shape (resembling the organ it would heal) or by color, the beet because of its redness, was good for the blood. It does contain some iron in a natural form which makes it easier to assimilate, but it is not the best source of that mineral.

Amino acids are present in good quantity, as well as the salts of phosphorus, sodium, calcium, potassium and magnesium. While the minerals are concentrated by cooking, the vitamins, including vitamins A, B-complex and C, are lost; so for therapy, it is best to use the raw juice. One glass alone or in a mixture once a day is the usual therapeutic dose. If taken in larger quantities it may cause dizziness or nausea. A combination of beet juice and carrot juice furnishes a good percentage combination of phosphorus, sulfur and potassium as well as a high concentration of vitamin A. An excellent toner and builder.

BRUSSELS SPROUTS

Botanical Origin: *Brassica oleracea variety gemmifera*

This "new" vegetable—it's only been around about 400 years—is a member of the cabbage family. The vegetable resembles a miniature cabbage and is descended from the wild cabbage, thanks to the skill of early Dutch gardeners.

These little cabbages are very important nutritionally because they have a long season—and, indeed, a little frost may improve the flavor—and are one of the top sources of vitamin C. A cupful of raw sprouts will contain 100 mg of vitamin C, which is twice the content of an equal weight of oranges. If that same cupful is cooked the vitamin C content will drop to 35 mg— another plug for raw juice.

According to many nutritionists, a combination of the juice of brussels sprouts, string beans, lettuce and carrot furnishes the elements needed to strengthen and regenerate the insulin-producing capacity of the pancreas. This combination, plus a diet which eliminates all concentrated starches and sugars, has been of value in cases of diabetes.

CABBAGE

Botanical Origin: *Brassica oleracea variety capit. alb.*

Cabbage, in contrast to its recently developed relative brussels sprouts, is one of the oldest vegetables known. It has been cultivated for over four thousand years. The cabbage family includes brussels sprouts, cauliflower, broccoli and kale. Cabbages themselves are either hard-head or loose-head, round-head, ovoid, flat or pointed, red or white.

Cabbage is loaded with vitamins and other nutrients. It combats nutritional deficiencies, boosts energy, improves chemical reactions within the body and is one of the most beneficial foods known to man.

Cabbage contains high levels of sulfur, calcium, phosphorus and iodine.

Its high level of vitamin A aids in tissue nutrition and rejuvenation.

The vitamin B1 content works to improve nerve function, the absorption of oxygen, and the metabolism of carbohydrates.

The vitamin B2 assists cellular chemical action.

The sulfur content combats infection and protects the skin against eczema.

Its magnesium, potassium and calcium help defend against illness.

The chlorophyll in cabbage helps to prevent anemia as long as the cabbage is eaten raw. Cooking destroys this factor.

The iron and copper build blood cells.

The protein and carbohydrate content build strong tissue and provide energy.

Duodenal ulcers have been soothed with cabbage juice. When the production of gas is too great, mix with carrot juice with a drop of cucumber juice for equal success. If the gas remains excessive it might indicate that the intestinal tract needs a cleaning. Try a combination of carrot and spinach juice daily for two or three weeks and then back to the cabbage juice.

Don't add salt and don't cook it. One hundred pounds of cooked cabbage will not supply the nutrients in 8 ounces of raw cabbage juice.

There are unknown factors in cabbage still to be identified. Because of its success in treating ulcers, one of the factors has been called vitamin U. Other factors have been known to act as natural antibiotics providing improved resistance to infection. Even sauerkraut, when prepared naturally, is of great benefit. Its fermentation aids in the digestion of cellulose and fats and makes it easily tolerated by the intestinal tract. Lactic acid, produced during fermentation, helps to disinfect the entire system.

This natural food, in balance with nature, seems superior to many compounds from the laboratory. Granted, it doesn't have the best taste in the world but mix it with carrot juice or add a bit of lemon or garlic and take one glass a day.

CARROT

Botanical Origin: *Daucus carota*

The ancient Greeks called the carrot *philon*, because they would eat the root as an aphrodisiac before making love. The root (*word* root this time) comes from *philo*, meaning love. The modern name comes from the Latin *carota*, which means, to burn, probably because of the reddish color. Carrots belong to the same family as celery, parsnips, caraway and dill and grow in all sizes and shapes from a bulbous red-purple beet-like root to pale yellow or white spheres. We are most familiar with the Mediterranean type, which is fairly long and deep yellow or orange in color.

Before we begin to investigate all the healthful properties of the carrot, let me put in a good word for the greens. Eat them raw—well washed, of course—in salads or add them last to soup because they have a lot of phosphorus and are helpful for nerve energy. Don't throw them away!

Don't scrape away the skin of the carrot before juicing. Wash it in running water and scrub it with a brush. Drink a pint a day since it can help normalize the entire system.

Principal constituents:

> *Vitamin A.* Actually it is a precursor called beta-carotene that the body can convert to vitamin A. Diabetics may have trouble with this conversion and frequently have to take vitamin A derived from fish liver oil.
> *Vitamins B-complex,* C, D, E and K.
> *Mineral salts* including iron (about 7 percent), calcium, sodium, potassium, magnesium, manganese, sulfur, copper, phosphorus.

Carrot juice provides energy; is a good source of minerals; helps to promote normal elimination; aids diuresis; helps to build healthy tissue and skin; stimulates appetite; helps build healthy teeth; helps prevent infections in the eyes and mucous membrane; contributes to the general health of the optic system; helps in the treatment of ulcers; furnishes vital enzymes to all body tissue.

The addition of a little cream (not milk) to carrot juice will result in an exotic flavor guaranteed to confuse most people who won't drink vegetable juice. Don't tell them, just heal them!

CHERRIES

Botanical Origin: *Amygdala Amara (sour)*
Amygdala Dulcis (sweet)

Prehistoric inhabitants of Europe and Asia left cherry pits in their cliff caves as did the ancient people of the Americas. The modern cherry probably originated in China, traveled to Italy and then to England. It arrived in America aboard the *Mayflower* and has been cultivated here ever since.

There are two basic types: the sweet cherry, about six hundred varieties, including the Queen Anne and the Bing, is larger than the sour cherry and needs a temperate climate. The sour cherry is cultivated in about three hundred forms.

Cherries have been used to alleviate the discomfort of gout and arthritis with much recorded success. Eat or juice a handful twice a day.

CELERY

Botanical Origin: *Apium graveolens*

Homer mentioned *selinon* in the *Odyssey*; it was probably celery or its close relative, parsley. It's difficult to separate the two historically, since they were both called by the same name. It was used as a diuretic and a laxative, to heal wounds, to soothe irritated nerves and to break up gallstones, and that was in the Middle Ages!

Today it is considered very helpful for diseases of

chemical imbalance and arthritis.

It contains vitamins A, B-complex and C as well as a lot of sodium and good amounts of magnesium, manganese, iron, iodine, copper, potassium, calcium and phosphorus.

There are important concentrations of plant hormones and essential oils which give celery its strong, characteristic smell. These oils have an effect on the regulation of the nervous system, seeming to calm a jittery state.

Celery also has been used for its stimulating effect upon the sexual system. It is particularly useful for a weak sex drive and those with normal sex drives can eat celery without fearing they will go off on a rampage— plant therapy tends to normalize a system!

Celery juice plus honey, one tablespoon to an 8-ounce glass, will help a dieter eat less if sipped slowly before a meal. It also makes a great and tasty drink on any occasion, and, before bedtime, a relaxing tonic.

CHARD

Botanical Origin: *Beta vulgaris cicla Chenopodiaceae*
Common Name: *Seakale Beet*

Often called Swiss Chard, it is actually a white-rooted beet. The root is not fleshy like other beets, and it is cultivated, not for the root, but for the leaves which are eaten like spinach and the stalks which are consumed like asparagus.

Most chard is green but there is a red variety now being cultivated in the United States.

Chard contains vitamins A and C as well as quantities

of iron. It has been used to build energy, as a laxative and as a diuretic.

The juice, mixed with carrot juice, has been used to help overcome urinary tract infections, constipation, hemorrhoids and certain skin diseases.

CHERVIL

Botanical Origin: *Cerefolium sativum*
Chaerophyllum sativum
Umbelliferae

Little known but very useful, chervil contains vitamins A and C, iron, and an estrogenic principal. Its list of benefits is long:

> provides energy
> promotes normal elimination
> aids diuresis
> stimulates the appetite
> enhances digestion
> stimulates the flow of bile
> combats diseases of the eye.

A juice prepared with chervil, wild chicory, lettuce and dandelion—equal parts of each—has been used for liver and gallbladder disease.

Two drops of fresh chervil juice in each eye three times a day relieves eye inflammation. (Check with your doctor before using.)

If you have ants in your closet, leave some pieces of chervil around and they'll soon depart for other, more pleasant areas.

COMFREY

Botanical Origin: *Symphytum officinale*

Comfrey has been used as a medicine since the time of ancient Greece. It was incorporated into an ointment and used to heal wounds and ulcers.

The active ingredient is allantoin, which is a cell proliferant and healing agent, stimulating healthy tissue growth. Modern therapy uses comfrey for its vitamin B12 content. It and alfalfa are the only land plants that can supply this much-needed vitamin. Vegetarians can obtain B12 without having to resort to animal foods and prevent the possible onset of anemia.

The juice is used for its valuable vitamin content and for its protein content, which is important in the cases of ulcers, fractures and wounds.

CUCUMBER

Botanical Origin: *Cucumis sativus*
Cucumis melo Cucurbitaceae

The cucumber originated in India. There is some mention of it as an emblem of fertility. One Buddhist legend tells about Sagara's wife who had 60,000 off-spring, the first of which was a cucumber who climbed to heaven on its own vine.

"As cool as a cucumber" is a factual description, since the interior temperature of a cucumber can be as much as twenty degrees cooler than the outside air on a warm day. Its cooling and thirst-quenching properties have been greatly appreciated by many hot and parched persons finding themselves in a cucumber garden. It contains more nature-distilled water than any other vegetable except the melon.

Cucumbers are very low in calories, about 3 calories to the ounce, hence those little cucumber sandwiches for dieters.

Cucumber is probably the best natural diuretic known. It has many other valuable properties, such as the promotion of hair growth due to its high silicon and sulfur content. Mix cucumber juice with carrot, lettuce and spinach juice.

Cucumber and carrot juice has been used for rheumatic ailments caused by an excess of uric acid in the system. Adding a little beet juice to the mixture helps speed up the cure.

Nails and hair respond well to cucumber juice therapy because of the combination of nutrients present. They are vitamins A, B-complex, and C as well as silicon, sulfur, manganese, lime, potassium, sodium, calcium and phosphorus.

CURRANT (Black)

Botanical Origin: *Ribes nigrum*

CURRANT (Red)

Botanical Origin: *Ribes rubrum*

Fresh currants are berries, in the same family as gooseberries. Dried currants are not currants at all but raisins made from the small, seedless grapes of Corinth.

Black currants are found mostly in northern Europe and Asia. They are the basis for a liqueur called cassis. Red currants are more common in the United States. There are also white currants, but they are really of the red variety which have lost their pigment.

Currants are rich in vitamin C, protein, carbohydrates, phosphorus, chlorine, sodium, potassium, magnesium and calcium. They also contain malic acid, emulsin and pectin.

Black currant syrup can be prepared as follows:

> Mix 1 kg of very ripe black currants,
>   2 grams of cinnamon,
>   12 grams of cloves.
> Let soak in 3 quarts of brandy containing 750 grams of brown sugar.
> Stir daily for one month, then mash the currants, strain and bottle.

An anti-arthritic tea is made as follows:

Black currant leaves	100 grams
Ash leaves	50 grams
Meadowsweet flowers	50 grams

Put one tablespoonful of the mixture in a glass and add 1 cup of boiling water. Let steep for fifteen minutes, then drink. Use three or four times a day.

Red currant juice is an appetite stimulant, a digestive aid, a laxative, a diuretic and a general body cleanser. The nutrients are about the same as in the black currant.

DANDELION

Botanical Origin: *Taraxacum officinale*

That yellow flower growing wild along the road, the bane of the green lawn, the weed in the garden, is an important vegetable. Not the flower but the leaves. They are bitter when eaten in a salad but can be steamed with something like sorrel.

If the need arose, a whole meal could be made of the dandelion. The roots steamed and buttered like parsnips, the crown and leaf stems could be a salad, and the whole could be washed down with dandelion wine.

Nutritionally, the dandelion is of remarkable value, containing as much iron as spinach, four times the vitamin A of lettuce, plus rich supplies of magnesium, potassium, calcium, sodium and vitamin C. It also contains quantities of folic acid, B-complex, silica, chlorophyll, and many other nutrients. The readily available organic magnesium makes the juice very valuable for all bone disorders. It is often mixed with the juice of carrots and turnips.

Dandelion juice is one of the most valuable tonics. It is used to counteract hyperacidity and to help normalize the system. The fresh juice is superior to tablets or capsules because it supplies the nutrients in a natural, organic form without added fillers or inorganic salts. All chemical magnesium preparations must take a back seat to the elements found in raw juice.

ENDIVE

Botanical Origin: *Cichorium endivia*

Also known as escarole and chicory, although there is some confusion. What we call endive is actually the leaf of the French *chicoree frisée*, and the curly-leaved chicory is actually an endive (or is it the other way 'round?).

In any case it is somewhat bitter, and the leaves are used for salads. It produces a blue flower somewhat like a dandelion with petals resembling the rays of the sun. Myth has it that Florilor, a beautiful lady, rejected the sun god's love because it did not include a proposal of marriage. Angered, he turned her into a flower whose rays mimic the sun. Perhaps that is the reason the seeds have been used since ancient times as a love potion.

Endive has elements needed by the optic system. A combination of the juice of endive with carrot, celery and parsley, one to two pints daily, have brought about fantastic vision improvement according to a number of people who have tried this combination.

Endive is the richest source of vitamin A among the green vegetables. It has been used in cases of hay fever, asthma and also for both liver and gallbladder dysfunction.

FENNEL

Botanical Origin: *Foeniculum vulgare, dulce*
Common Name: *Finocchio*

Fennel is the basis for anise, and flavors some brandy-based drinks. The leaves are an important culinary additive. In the Middle Ages it was noted that insects disliked fennel so the stalks were spread on the floors to keep away fleas and other crawlies. Fennel was used to plug up keyholes so the night demons could not enter and on Midsummer Eve a wreath of fennel kept the witches quiet.

Fennel is related to celery, and contains an essential oil that soothes an irritated stomach. The juice of fennel combined with carrot juice is a tonic for the eyes and, when beet juice is added is helpful for anemia caused by excessive menstrual flow.

Its main ingredients are vitamins A, B-complex and C, and minerals, including calcium and phosphorus, sulfur, iron and potassium. Fennel juice helps digest a meal of beans and lima beans and reduces the flatulence which usually follows.

FIGS

Botanical Origin: *Ficus carica*

The most familiar reference to figs is in the Bible when Adam and Eve sewed fig leaves together to make an apron. Fig leaves are thin and the texture is quite rough and altogether unsuitable for an apron or any other piece of clothing, but I guess we have to allow for biblical license. In any event, the fig is one of the oldest fruits known to man. Fossil figs have been found in caves dating back some 65 million years.

The fig is an easily digestible, healthful food, a good source of energy and a collection of great nutritional values.

Figs contain:

> vitamins A, B-complex and C.
> minerals, including iron, manganese, calcium and bromine.
> enzymes including amylase and protease.

Figs are used to correct constipation in the form of juice or syrup—and, if you're lucky enough to have fig leaves, they're wonderful for cleaning pots and pans.

GOOSEBERRY

Botanical Origin: *Ribes uva-crispa*

This is a new fruit, only cultivated for about a hundred years. The skin is fairly translucent and feels slightly fuzzy. It may be red or green or a yellowish-white in color. The leaves are often used in salads.

As are most fruits, the gooseberry is a source of vitamins A, B-complex and C, and the minerals potassium, calcium, iron, bromine and phosphorus.

Benefits:

> has been used to promote appetite
> aid digestion
> promote normal bowel function
> promote diuresis
> supply vitamin C
> supply important minerals.

If you can find gooseberries, juice about a double handful and divide it into three doses. Take the first glass before eating breakfast.

GRAPE

Botanical Origin: *Vitis vinifera Ampelideae*

Adam and Eve and Noah planted grapes, and all grapes have descended from the original vines. Grapes are red, black, green or white, seedless or seeded. The natural blending of acid, natural sugar, mucilage, and bitter and astringent properties make the juice acceptable to even the most delicate stomach. In some health spas, cures are effected with a diet of bread and grapes and nothing else except pure spring water.

Grapes contain vitamins, minerals, malic acid, fermentable sugar, free acids, tannin, volatile acid and water.

Grapes are easily digested, and:

> are a superior energy source
> are a superior mineral source
> build a healthy skin
> enhance normal bowel function
> improve urinary flow.

The health spa grape cure promotes diuresis, and enhances bile flow and normal elimination. It is indicated for dyspepsia, constipation and other conditions. The technique is to take 700 to 1400 grams of juice without taking any other food.

Since this is basically a juice-fasting technique, it should not be undertaken without medical advice.

GRAPEFRUIT

Botanical Origin: *Citrus decumana putaceae*

The fruit grows in clusters, and if a person was very nearsighted, the cluster might look like a bunch of grapes and that is perhaps how it got its name—which could also be a corruption of "Greatfruit," from its size.

It is a good appetizer and

> aids digestion
> promotes normal flow of urine
> helps to remove impurities from the blood.

Grapefruit contains citric acid, sugars, pectins, essential oils including limonene, pinene and citral, plus vitamins C, calcium, phosphorus, vitamin A and vitamin P.

Some people have tried to diet by eating nothing but grapefruit or by drinking the juice without any other food. This is, of course, another version of a juice fast and cannot present the body with balanced nutrition. Most people can fast for three days without any side effects, but to do it without supervision for more than three days is foolhardy.

LEMON

Botanical Origin: *Citrus limonia*

The brighter the lemon and the better it looks, the more you should wash it with soap and water if you intend to use the peel. Some lemons are waxed to improve their appearance and others are dipped in a chemical. Play safe and wash them.

The pulp left after juicing is excellent for the skin and takes the pain away from insect bites. Add a little glycerine to the pulp for a great hand lotion to keep the skin smooth. (Readers who saw the movie *Atlantic City* will be vividly aware of this property.)

Acid predominates in the lemon, one ounce of juice containing forty grains of citric acid. Many home remedies include lemon, for example:

Colds and coughs: drink juice straight or mixed with another juice.

Fever: lemon promotes perspiration and heating lemon helps to form salicylic acid, which is a pain-killer.

Indigestion: lemon juice with a bit of salt taken after meals.

Reducing diet: mix lemon juice and barley water and drink before meals.

Skin and scalp problems: lemon juice rubbed into the scalp against dandruff.

Warts and corns: for warts, steep the rind in vinegar, then rub on; for corns, use the juice alone.

Rheumatism: mix the juice with a pinch of powdered garlic and drink it on an empty stomach.

LETTUCE

Botanical Origin: *Lactuca sativa*
Lactuca virosa Compositae

Edible lettuce is a relative of poison lettuce, a common European plant. Most lettuce is potentially narcotic and, for this reason, was known as "sleepwort" to the Anglo-Saxons. The dried juice from the wild lettuce was used as a sedative and hypnotic and mixed with honey as a cough suppressor. Possibly lettuce in the wild contains an ingredient that has these effects.

Cultivated lettuce has great quantities of iron and magnesium. Magnesium salts need calcium to operate efficiently, and lettuce contains calcium also, as well as a wonderful blend of other minerals. They include iodine, phosphorus, copper, cobalt, zinc and potassium.

The vitamin content includes a great deal of provitamin A, but bear in mind that the outer green leaves can contain as much as fifty times more nutrients than the inner white leaves—so juice *everything*. Don't soak lettuce in water. Many of the water-soluble vitamins will be lost. Rinse it to get rid of any dirt, but do not soak.

Many of the therapeutic effects are due to the alkaloids present. They include asparagine, lactucine, lactucuc acid and hyoscyamine. There is also a large chlorophyll content, particularly in the outside green leaves. Other vitamins present are vitamins C, D, E and B-complex.

Even though most hair loss is genetically induced, there is some loss due to faulty nutrition. A daily drink of a pint of lettuce juice combined with carrot and spinach juice is said to furnish food to the scalp nerves and roots of the hair. Or you might alternate by mixing lettuce juice with carrot, green pepper and fresh alfalfa juice. This mixture is also said to help hair return to its original color.

Romaine lettuce is different chemically from head lettuce. The juice of Romaine lettuce, when combined with a small amount of kelp (seaweed), has been said to help the functions of the adrenal gland. Romaine is rich in sodium, nearly 60 percent more than its potassium content. This proportion is valuable in certain disease states.

NETTLE

Botanical Origin: *Urtica dioica et urens*

The stinging nettle lends itself more to herbology than to regular juice therapy, although there is a fine distinction, since the juice of herbs can be called juice therapy. Perhaps the biggest difference is that many herbal extracts are made with boiling water or with extracts of alcohol-soluble ingredients, while juicing just separates the natural juice from the pulp.

The juice will help bleeding in the mouth. Taken three times a day, a tablespoonful at a time, it is useful for hemorrhoids.

The active ingredients are:

> formic acid
> histamine
> gallic acid

plus a large quantity of organic iron which makes nettle juice very useful in cases of anemia.

It is a diuretic for the kidneys and helps eliminate uric acid.

MELON

Botanical Origin: *Cucumis melo cucurbitaceae*

Melons belong to the same family as cucumbers and

squash. They are usually eaten raw and they are the most cooling fruit around. In the tropics or in areas where the water is not the safest fluid to drink, melons provide a tasty alternative. You can store a melon and change it into a canteen by punching a hole in it and then plugging it up with wax or a cork if you have one handy. After a few days most of the flesh will have liquified into a delightful drink. For those who like an alcoholic beverage, pour in a bit of wine or brandy before you seal it.

Melons are good tonics and assist in elimination. When combined with lemon juice, they are supposed to help eliminate excess uric acid. Melons contain sugar, cellulose, vitamins A, B1 and C.

MULBERRY

Botanical Origin: *Morus nigra moraceae*

Pyramus and Thisbe met secretly under a white mulberry tree, and it was the scene of their tragic end. When Thisbe plunged the sword into her breast her blood spouted over the tree and the fruit was stained red forever more.

Well, not quite!

The white mulberry is actually one of the most important tree plants because it is the tree upon whose leaves the silkworm feeds.

The natural benefits of the black mulberry are as follows:

> a bracing tonic
> aids elimination

contains vitamin A and C
contains tannin, an astringent.

ORANGE

Botanical Origin: *Citrus sinensis*

The name may have come from the French word for
gold, or obviously because of the fruit's color and taste.
Orange blossoms are still worn by brides because the
god Jupiter gave an orange to Juno when they were
married. Oranges have been called the "apples of the
sun." The oil of the orange is highly aromatic and is
called oil of neroli.

All oranges are tree-ripened and many, despite what
we think, are ripe when they are green. Oranges will
not ripen after being picked, the way some foods will. A
temperature drop can cause an "orange" orange to turn
green. Some pickers will take green oranges and treat
them with ethylene to decompose the chlorophyll and
turn it orange. Others do that and then add dye and
wax, all that so the fruit will be more physically appealing. So, beware of perfect-looking oranges. If they have
green spots they are probably more natural.

Oranges are either sweet or sour. Sweet oranges are
more popular for juicing while sour oranges are mostly
for making marmalade. There is one orange that is
grown for the oil that can be extracted. It is called the
Bergamot orange and the oil is used for making per-
fume and soap.

Oranges, when ripe, will have some 50 mg to 100 mg
of vitamin C per each 100 mg of fruit (a small orange).
It also has a quantity of bioflavonoids (vitamin P) which
is Nature's special ally of vitamin C. Bioflavonoids are

found in many vitamin C-rich fruits such as rosehips, green peppers, and strawberries. Alone or in combination they have been used as anticoagulants, for capillary fragility, and for the treatment of colds. A glass of juice daily can be a good source of vitamin C.

The principal constituents found in oranges are:

water	90%
carbohydrates	5.6%
acid	2.5%
protein	.7%
cellulose	1%
vitamins B1, B2, C, P	
carotene	
mineral salts: iron, calcium, potassium, magnesium, phosphorus, sodium, copper, zinc, manganese and bromine.	

PAPAYA

Botanical Origin: *Carica papaya*

The papaya is a treasure house of proteolytic enzymes, the chemicals that make digestion easy. Papain is the most important of these enzymes, and it is extracted from the papaya and then dried into a powder form for use as a digestant. It is also used as a meat tenderizer to partially break down meat fibers.

Papaya juice can be used by people with poor digestive ability. Older people in particular may be not digesting food properly, thereby not obtaining the nutrients needed for the proper function of the body.

Papaya juice used on a regular basis can mark a turning point in how they digest and assimilate food and how they feel in general.

If the main purpose of juicing is to improve digestion, buy the papaya while it is still green. The unripe fruit contains more of the enzyme than the ripened one.

Papaya also contains fibrin, which is a very rare thing for a plant product, since it is usually only found in animals and in man. In man it is part of the blood-clotting process. It also contains arginine, thought to be good for male fertility, and carpain, an enzyme thought to be helpful for the heart.

Papaya contains high levels of vitamins A and C, very little fat, and a bit of protein. A wonderfully therapeutic digestive drink can be made by combining papaya with pineapple juice which contains another digestive enzyme called bromelain. As a juice, this combination can be useful for almost every type of affliction.

PARSLEY

Botanical Origin: *Petroselinum sativum*
Apium petroselinum
Carum petroselinum

Parsley, garlic, dandelion, carrot and leek are our leading vegetable medical remedies. Parsley contains three times as much vitamin C as does the orange. It also contains as much vitamin A as the carrot. So why do we push it aside when it is put on our plate to provide a green contrast? It is more than a garnish, it is a powerful source of nutrients.

Parsley is an herb. The juice is very strong and rarely should be taken alone. Mix one ounce with at least four onces of carrot juice.

Parsley contains:

> vitamins A, B-complex and C
> estrogens
> chlorophyll
> enzymes
> minerals: iron, calcium, phosphorus, magnesium, sulfur, potassium, iodine, copper and manganese
> essential oils: pinene, terpene, apiol, apein.

Parsley can affect oxygen metabolism, the urinary tract, the capillary system, the eyes and optic nerve system (particularly when mixed with carrot, celery and endive), the adrenal and the thyroid glands.

Cramps associated with menstrual problems have been relieved by regular use of this juice when concentrated starches and sugars have been eliminated from the diet along with the use of the juice.

Dried parsley is not a satisfactory alternative. It would be better to freeze fresh parsley and then use it in soups or gravies.

The body can be in desperate need of potassium and all the other organic minerals. It is one of the wonders of the plant world that it can reach down into the soil and extract inorganic minerals that we could not assimilate in our bodies, and turn them into organic, living salts we can use easily. A raw vegetable combination of parsley juice, carrot juice, celery juice and spinach juice can supply practically all of the minerals needed.

It is not as tasty as some of the other juice combinations but it is jammed full of health. Convalescents should sip a glass a day to speed up recovery since these minerals are needed for the regeneration of cells and tissue. There is no drug available that can do what plain, raw vegetable juice can do.

PARSNIP

Botanical Origin: *Pastinaca sativa*

The parsnip has usually been used for soups along with onions, potatoes and leeks. It is very low in calories, which makes it ideal as a soup for persons wanting to lose weight.

It has been used as a diuretic, an anti-arthritic and a detoxifying agent.

The juice is low in calcium but rich in potassium, phosphorus, sulfur, silicon and chlorine. Don't confuse the organic chlorine, which is important to the body, with the chlorine used as a disinfectant. It contains the rare combination of sulfur and silicon which is helpful to the strength and growth of nails and hair. Parsnip juice is particularly valuable in the case of brittle nails. A daily juice drink plus a weekly buffing with a nail buffer should restore the nail to health in a very short time.

The juice has also been helpful to people with an assortment of lung problems. It seems the unique combination of chlorine and phosphorus is helpful in those conditions.

Do not pick parsnips in the woods and take them home for use either in the juicer or in making soup. Wild parsnips may have some poisonous ingredients. Buy only the cultivated variety.

PEACHES *Prunus Persica*

PEARS *Pyrus Communis*

PERSIMMONS *Diospyros Virginiana/ Diospyros Kaki*

PLANTAINS *Musa Paradisiaca*

PLUMS *Prunus Proumnon*

What's the use of making up a format for a book if you can't change it once in a while? The fruits listed above are seldom juiced at home but eaten whole. That the juice is digested more quickly without the pulp will not make a lot of difference to the reader, because it is so enjoyable to eat these fruits just as they come from Nature. However, I feel it's important to know as much as possible, even if you don't juice these.

Peaches originated in China and then were transported and grown all over the world wherever they would root and grow fruit. Columbus carried peach seeds on his voyages. Peaches and almonds make great friends and almond kernels impregnated with peach pollen often produce peaches. The oil from the peach pit is used for soap manufacture and as a substitute for almond oil. An infusion of the leaves and bark is used for treating gastritis, cough and chronic bronchitis.

Pears also originated in Asia and were cultivated by the Chinese. There are more than three thousand varieties of pear, although only about twenty varieties are popular. Pears can be made into cider much like apples and it is excellent to drink.

Two to three glasses of the juice may be taken daily. It contains vitamins A, B1, B2, P and C. Also the minerals phosphorus, sodium, calcium, magnesium, sulfur, potassium, chlorine, copper, manganese and iodine.

Persimmons have an irritating astringency unless they are fully ripe. The astringency is due to a large amount of tannic acid in the fruit. They are also rich in pepsin, which is an aid to digestion.

Plantains look like bananas but are longer, thicker, more starchy and not as sweet. They are not eaten raw as the banana is, but are cooked or roasted. In that way they are more vegetable than fruit.

Plums are blue, red, yellow, green and combinations of them all. All prunes are plums but not all plums can become prunes. A specific type of plum tree produces the fruit that can be dried without fermenting and still contain the pit. The Huns, Turks, Mongols and Tartars used these dried plums as a nutritious part of their diet because they could carry a large quantity around with their armies and not depend on the land they were fighting on to supply them with food. Prunes are natural laxatives because of their high cellulose content and also help to eliminate mucus because of their acid content.

PINEAPPLE

Botanical Origin: *Ananas sativus*

Pineapple contains the protein digestant called bromelain. It is comparable in potency with pepsin and papain and can digest 1,000 times its weight in protein.

Since it is available on a year-round basis, fresh pineapple is a useful provider of vitamin C during the winter when other fresh fruits are hard to obtain. The juice helps relieve the discomfort of a sore throat and bronchitis and helps dissolve mucus formations, and aids the function of the kidney. When buying pineapples look for a good color since pineapples do not continue to ripen once they've been removed from the stem.

Pineapples contain vitamins A, B-complex and C plus the minerals iodine, magnesium, manganese, potassium, calcium, phosphorus, iron and sulfur. They also provide citric and malic acids.

Canned juice, even if there is no added sugar, loses two-thirds of its nutritional value.

POTATO

Botanical Origin: *Solanum tuberosum*

There is no more important vegetable than the potato. Millions of people have survived during periods of famine because the potato was available. When first brought to Europe, it was thought to be poisonous—it is indeed related to the deadly nightshade and under certain conditions can be dangerous—but this tuber is linked to man and has influenced his life.

Potatoes can be baked, broiled, boiled, fried and mashed and can be considered the perfect meal when eaten with herring, or so say the Irish. In truth, the combination does supply vitamins A, B, C and D, mineral salts, carbohydrate, protein and fats which is a fairly complete meal.

The poisonous parts of the potato are not in the potato itself—that is the part of the plant below the ground—it is the parts above the ground that are dangerous: the flower, leaf, stem and berry, which contain solanine. If there are any green spots on the potato, remove them before using, and remove any shoots that may appear. Store potatoes in a cool, dark place.

Now, what about potato juice? It is perfectly drinkable as it comes from the juicer, but its taste and effect are improved by adding lemon or carrot juice. The juice is very soothing to the stomach and useful in cases of ulcers and gastritis.

It is also very cleansing to the system. When combined with carrot and celery, it has been used for gout.

Potatoes are important enough to give a complete rundown of the constituents:

water	75%
carbohydrates	22%
protein	2%
lipids	.14%
mineral salts	1.05%

sodium, calcium, magnesium, phosphorus, iron, manganese, copper and sulfur quantities of vitamins B-complex, C, K, folic acid, pantothenic acid.

Don't be influenced by the stories that potatoes are fattening, because they're not. They are a wonderful food. Juice them or eat them baked—just don't put on the butter and salt!

RADISH

Botanical Origin: *Raphanus niger (black)*
Raphanus sativus (pink)

Pictures of the radish are carved on the Egyptian temples at Karnak. The builders must have munched on this pungent vegetable as they plied their trade. A statue of a radish stood in the temple at Delphi, made of solid gold. Later, the radish was used to cure madness, detect witches, cause demons to leave a body they wanted to possess, make people think and speak with wit, and cure headache and shingles. This is the background of that vegetable we frequently see carved into pretty rosettes on a bed of lettuce . . . and leave aside on the plate.

Radishes are very good for the body. They have a high alkali content and benefit the kidney and bladder. They also contain a good supply of sulfur and phosphorus.

You can make an interesting juice by combining three radishes, one-half onion and pineapple juice. Try it.

The black radish contains vitamins B1, C and E and some sulfur compounds, while the pink radish contains vitamins B-complex, C, D and P, plus a sulfur compound, magnesium and iodine, as well as a large amount of potassium and sodium.

The juice should never be taken alone; it's much too strong. It can be mixed with carrot juice to help restore the tone of the mucous membrane.

RHUBARB

Botanical Origin: *Rheum officinale*
Rheum palmatum

Rhubarb is not a friend to man. I was tempted to leave it out of the book altogether, but that would not have been fair to all the people who have been told about its nutritional value.

It does have some benefits, but these are offset by one constituent that can cause trouble. That is the high oxalic acid content. Few plants have as much oxalic acid as rhubarb. When cooked, this acid is converted into an inorganic chemical which deposits oxalic acid crystals in the body. Rhubarb does have a laxative effect and people have used it as a laxative without giving thought to the side effects of the deposited oxalic acid.

Some benefit can be obtained from drinking raw rhubarb juice in small quantities. It will increase peristalsis and stimulate a bowel movement. Sweeten the juice with a little honey to make it more palatable.

What I have said refers to the underground stems; the leaves should not be used *at all*.

SPINACH

Botanical Origin: *Spinacia oleracea*

Spinach is a member of the goosefoot family, and many of its relatives are weeds. Most of us remember overcooked spinach, a green mess, soft and soggy and a thing to be avoided. That's unfortunate, because it is a nutritious food when eaten raw or lightly steamed—and it actually tastes good!

Some nutritionists play down the use of spinach because they say it has an oxalic acid content that will interfere with the calcium content, making it insoluble and therefore of no use to the body. However, there are so many other nutrients that spinach should be a part of the diet.

Spinach is excellent for the intestinal tract. Raw spinach juice, about one pint a day, will correct the most stubborn case of constipation.

Spinach contains:

> Vitamins A, B-complex, C, folic acid, sodium, potassium, calcium, iron, phosphorus, magnesium, sulfur, manganese, zinc, copper, iodine, chlorophyll and mucilage.

It is not recommended for people with a tendency to kidney stones, because of the oxalic acid content, but is recommended for all others.

STRAWBERRY

Botanical Origin: *Fragaria vesca rosaceae*

What would you say about a medicine if you saw it advertised in a drugstore window as follows:

> Aids defense against disease
> Can be used as a laxative
> Can promote normal urinary production
> Combats gout by promoting the elimination of

uric acid
Helps to lower blood pressure
Promotes normal metabolism of the liver, endocrine glands and the nervous system
Has astringent properties when applied to the skin
And it is a tasty energy-providing nutrient

You would call it a miracle drug!

But that is what many nutritionists say are the natural benefits of the strawberry.

It contains vitamins B-complex, C, E, K plus iron, sodium, phosphorus, magnesium, potassium, sulfur, calcium, silicon, iodine and bromine. Since the carbohydrate in strawberries is levulose, it may be acceptable for diabetics. Check with the doctor first.

TOMATO

Botanical Origin: *Lycopersicum esculentum*

Question: Is the tomato a fruit or a vegetable?
Answer: Neither, it is a berry!
However, in 1893 the Supreme Court of the United States officially designated it as a vegetable because fruits were allowed to be imported without duty.

Tomatoes, like the potato, are members of the deadly nightshade family, so for a good part of time they were only used for their decorative value. Far from being poisonous, tomatoes are rich in vitamin C and vitamin A. They are also rich in potassium. All this is true if tomatoes are allowed to ripen naturally. If they are picked green and allowed to ripen after harvesting, the nutritional content is much less. Cooking and canning reduces the value of the juice less than other juices, but canned juice still cannot compare to fresh. A mixture of carrot, spinach and tomato juices is used for anemic conditions, particularly for children who find the mixture an easy way to get organic iron.

Tomatoes contain: Vitamins A, B1, B2, B6, C and K, also iron, bromine and phosphorus.

TURNIP

Botanical Origin: *Brassica napus*
Brassica rapa

Turnips are not usually juiced. Yet, turnip leaves contain more calcium by percentage than any other vegetable. This makes it an excellent source of organic calcium for growing children and for anyone who suffers from bone softening in any form. Turnip leaf juice combined with carrot and dandelion juices supplies calcium and magnesium, plus potassium in the correct proportions to give teeth and bones the necessary hardness.

Turnips started out many centuries ago as field cabbage. During years of cultivation they retained their cabbage-like leaves but became rough and slightly hairy. They can be white, yellow, red, gray, long, round or flat.

Do not let the turnip top get away, because 90 percent of the nutrition resides there. The root is delicious as a vegetable if it is sautéed in a little oil or added to a stew. Some people like to use it raw in salads.

In addition to the splendid mineral content, turnip

juice also contains vitamins A, B-complex and C as well as magnesium, sulfur, iodine, iron and copper.

It is said that an eight-week diet of raw fruit and vegetables plus a daily tonic of the juice of carrot, spinach, watercress and turnip, will be found very effective in reducing hemorrhoids.

WATERCRESS

Botanical Origin: *Nasturtium officinale*

Watercress was used as a medicine before it became a food. The Persians believed it aided growth, the Romans thought it was effective against falling hair. Modern nutritionists now know that certain sulfur-bearing amino acids are necessary for the healthy growth of hair. Watercress contains more sulfur than any other vegetable except horseradish. Maybe the Romans had something when they ate watercress and bread.

There's also a good reason not to fight for a taxi with a little old lady who has just had her watercress sandwich. You might lose! In addition to the high sulfur content, watercress contains sodium, potassium, calcium and iron; and its vitamin content is high as well. Among the vitamins it can supply are valuable amounts of vitamin A (carotene), folic acid, biotin, nicotinic acid, pantothenic acid, vitamin B1, and large quantities of vitamin C. That's not all. If you need iodine for the correct functioning of the thyroid gland and you don't like sea vegetables like kelp, watercress is one of the best sources.

The juice is much too strong to take alone. Various mixtures lend themselves to various conditions. When

added to cucumber and beet juice it aids a gouty condition; with turnip top juice, carrot and spinach it builds
red blood; a mixture with potato, parsley and carrot
helps the lungs.

6. *How to Buy a Juicer*

::

WHAT IS an ideal juicer?

It will make the maximum amount of juice from a given quantity of any material. The residue will be rather dry and can be used on salads or in soups and gravies for its fiber content, or used in the garden as compost.

It is my opinion that blenders do not meet the need because they do not remove the solid factors present in fruits and vegetables. Blenders do serve a function, and I use a blender when I am not looking for therapeutic benefits. They're marvelous for making delicious fun drinks and for mixing juices once they have been separated from the solid material. The reason I'm harping on the separation of liquid from solid is that raw juices will be assimilated and be effective in about fifteen or twenty minutes after ingestion. If the solid portion is not separated from the juice, the stomach treats it as a regular food and digests it in the normal manner which may be a matter of hours.

For the purpose of juice therapy you must buy a juicing machine. They are not inexpensive, so you have to think a bit about what machine will do the best job for you. Some machines are better at one job but will have disadvantages of cleaning; others will have aluminum parts instead of stainless steel. Nutritionists tend to shy away from aluminum but they are less expensive and that may be an advantage. High-quality plastic is acceptable and is frequently combined with stainless steel.

Juice machines usually come with a one-year guarantee against any manufacturing fault. That's the least amount of time that I would find acceptable.

There are a number of basic types of machines. The simplest one can be likened to a basket with holes in it. The material is pressed against a cutter or cutters through a feeding hole. The material is divided into fine particles and whirled around at a great speed forcing the juice through tiny holes by centrifugal action. The solid material is retained in the basket while the juice comes out a spigot. This is a good machine, simple to use, but it must be emptied of the solid material after every pint or so. If this is difficult to do or if this makes the sink filthy or if it requires too much dexterity to disassemble and assemble all of the time, then you will not be inclined to use it, and all the benefits you might get will be lost. Before you buy, take the machine apart and put it back together. Try to see if you would use it daily, because it is daily use that'll make you healthy.

The next kind is called a continuous-action machine. The food is fed through a feeder against the rotating cutters and the juice comes out one end and the solid material, the other end. This is a convenient machine and will make a lot of juice at one time. If there is a problem it is that it doesn't seem to be as powerful at separating the juice from the fiber as the centrifugal machine. It is easy to feed the material into the machine and easy to empty the basket which holds the residue but, in some machines, the residue is deposited along the plastic guide which can be a bit messy.

VERY IMPORTANT: You must clean all machines

after every usage. Dirty machines will break down easily and the material left behind can cause odor or bacteria buildup. The machine has to be cleaned with soap and water, so that ease of assembly has to be considered. Frequently the difference in the cost of a machine may be found to be unimportant if you know you'll use it because it's easier.

If you're lucky enough to have inherited a small wine press, you've saved a lot of money. A wine press will give you a wonderful juice. Just take the fruit or vegetable. Cut it into small pieces and put it into the wine basket. Start turning the screw, which will force a plate against the material and the juice will start flowing. This is a simple, easy and long-lasting device.

The hydraulic press is an expensive cousin to the wine press. The pressure on the material can go up to 7,000 pounds and every last bit of juice is extracted. It is the most efficient means of obtaining juice, but it is a little cumbersome for apartment use unless you have a large family and a large, large kitchen. If you do and you can afford it, it is desirable.

Some food processors include a juicing attachment. If you need a machine that can do shredding, chopping, grinding and juicing, it may pay to look into their capabilities. I have not found them to be more than adequate as juicers—a bit like using the blender and ending up with a purée instead of juice. However, it's better to have a poor machine you'll use all of the time than a great machine gathering dust.

The following represents my experience with different machines. The results are strictly subjective, and I strongly suggest that you try any of these machines for yourself. What I like you may not like, and vice versa.

The Champion Juicer

This juicer is quite versatile with various attachments for a variety of preparations. It can juice, grate and homogenize. It is made of plastic and stainless steel. It is of the continuous extraction type. The material is fed onto a rotating cutter housed in an extension at the front of the machine. The juice comes out through a screen at the bottom of the extension while the pulp comes out through the front.

It is relatively easy to clean and there is not a lot of vibration. The manufacturer says it can be used to make grated vegetables, juices, nut butters, snow cones, ice cream, sherbet and baby food.

The Braun Juicer

This machine is of the centrifugal type. It extracts a great deal of juice and leaves a dry pulp. It is not difficult to take apart and clean. It should be cleaned after a pint or so of juice has been extracted and it's not for a large family. Some models vibrate a bit while they are working.

This machine is suitable for a working couple who will have a glass of juice each.

The Norwalk Hydraulic Press

This is the largest and heaviest machine for home use. It weighs 60 pounds, has a powerful half-horsepower motor, is guaranteed for two years, and does more things than any other machine. It's also the most expensive. If you're rich . . . look into this one!

It is a hydraulic press juicer, completely pulp free. It's a salad maker. It makes nut butters from nuts without adding oil. It's a flour mill. It's a coffee grinder. It's a dessert maker—shaved ice, snow cones, frozen fruit, etc.

This is not your typical home machine unless you live in a mansion, but it's a beauty.

The Phoenix Juicer

This machine is a continuous action machine pretty much like the one I described in the opening chapter. It is fairly easy to clean and will let you make a large quantity of juice at one time. Some models leave too much pulp in the juice, but the cost and the quantity of juice that can be made at one time may make up for that drawback. It does not have vibration problems and the noise level is low to moderate.

It can be used for a family of two, or a family of five or more, and juices fruits or vegetables, skin, pits and all.

Vitamix

This is a "total" juicer in that it reduces everything to a liquid, peels, seeds and all.

It is a soup maker (hot or cold), a bread dough mixer, a meat chopper, and a salad maker. It can make ice cream, nut butters, baby food, sherbets etc. It has a five-year replacement guarantee on parts.

It is a very versatile machine. Since it uses every part of the food, some of the product is a bit thick and requires the addition of some water as a dilutant.

The Omega Juicer

In writing this book, I tested many juicers—the good, the not-so-good and, just recently, what I consider to be the superb!

It is the American-made Omega Juicer, which comes with spinner basket, cutting blade and bowl, all made of pure stainless steel; a lid made of non-porous, non-formaldehyde, sturdy plastic; a long-lasting induction motor, permanently sealed bearings, and a hand-balanced basket and rotor for better stability.

I think this Omega Juicer is the best, most economical juicer to buy. It extracts 20–30 percent more juice than most other brands on the market. Its workmanship and ease of operation make it quick and easy to juice the nutritious fruits and vegetables that will reward you with continuing good health. I find the machine easy to clean and a sheer joy to use. And, as you would expect of a quality product, the Omega is backed by a full ten-year guarantee, parts *and* labor (except the blade, which has a one-year guarantee).

The Omega also has a nifty citrus attachment (optional) for making citrus juices quickly and easily, a pint in a minute or less.

Acme Juicerator

The Acme is a centrifugal juicer with a ten-year guarantee. It is easy to clean, and has very little vibration as it works.

7. *What and Why Are Those Wonderful Nutrients in Fruits and Vegetables?*

LIFE gives to life the nutrients needed to sustain it. The difference between organic (living) and inorganic (not living) is apparent. Anyone can point out the difference between life and death when it is gross, but our bodies can differentiate living and dead substances on the submolecular level. The body recognizes familiar molecules and incorporates them into its being. It rejects unfamiliar molecules and either destroys or expels them from the body.

Metallic zinc, as it comes from the earth, cannot be used by the body at all. As a matter of fact if it is ingested it will be poisonous. However, once it has been incorporated into the tissue of a plant, the gift of organic life is given to it and it can be utilized by the body for a number of very important reactions.

The same transmutation takes place with all the minerals, trace minerals, vitamins, enzymes, pro-vitamins etc., found in plant tissue. Whatever their role before they have been transformed by the plant, after the transformation they become useful to our bodies.

In what way are they useful? What functions do they perform? What do vitamins do? Why do we need minerals?

I'll give a brief explanation of the function of some of the nutrients found in food—not a complete explanation by any means but enough, I hope, to make you want to be sure you supply all of them to yourself and your family every day.

VITAMINS & ENZYMES

Vitamin A:
Also known as carotene. It is fat soluble, unstable in air, destroyed by ultraviolet light. It is essential for growth of young; increases resistance to urinary and respiratory infection; is necessary for lactation, reproduction, proper appetite and digestion; is necessary for vision, for the health of the skin and for the health of all mucous membranes.

Deficiency symptoms include: allergies, brittle hair, dry skin, fatigue, night blindness, poor appetite, poor digestion, retarded growth, sinus problems, sterility.

Vitamin B1:
Also known as thiamine hydrochloride. It is water-soluble, unstable in ultraviolet light, destroyed by heat; cannot be stored in the body, must be supplied daily; is necessary for absorption and digestion of food, blood building, carbohydrate metabolism. It corrects and prevents beri-beri, promotes growth, resistance to infection and proper nerve function.

Deficiency symptoms include: beri-beri, fatigue, intestinal disorders, irritability, numbness of hands and feet, poor lactation, poor appetite, shortness of breath, slow heart beat, ulcers, weakness.

Vitamin B2:
Also known as riboflavin. Water-soluble, cannot be stored in the body; necessary for antibody and red blood cell formation; aids in the assimilation of iron and protein

metabolism. Necessary for good vision, healthy skin and digestive tract.

Deficiency symptoms include: cataracts, digestive disturbance, hair loss, impaired lactation, lack of stamina, pellagra, retarded growth.

Vitamin B3:
Also known as niacin. Water-soluble, cannot be stored in the body; necessary for circulation, sex hormone production, growth, metabolism, respiration; helps to reduce cholesterol level.

Deficiency symptoms include: appetite loss, canker sores, depression, fatigue, halitosis, headaches, indigestion, insomnia, muscular weakness, nausea, nerve disorders, skin problems.

Vitamin B5:
Also known as pantothenic acid. Water-soluble, cannot be stored in the body; unstable to heat, destroyed by vinegar or baking soda; necessary for antibody formation, carbohydrate metabolism, growth, healthy skin and nerves; maintains blood sugar level, stimulates adrenal glands.

Deficiency symptoms include: adrenal exhaustion, depression, diarrhea, hair loss, hypoglycemia, intestinal disorders, kidney problems, premature aging, skin disorders.

Vitamin B6:
Also known as pyridoxine. Water-soluble, cannot be stored in the body; unstable in light or heat; necessary for antibody formation, controls levels of magnesium in the blood system and tissues, maintains sodium/potassium balance, aids digestion, metabolism of fats, cholesterol level.

Deficiency symptoms include: acne, anemia, arthritis, behavioral changes, dizziness, hair loss, irritability, learning disabilities, swelling, weakness.

Vitamin B12:
Also known as cyanocobalamin. Water-soluble, cannot be stored in the body; necessary for appetite, blood cell formation, cell longevity, normal metabolism of nerve tissue, protein, fat and carbohydrate metabolism, utilization of iron.

Deficiency symptoms include: menstrual disturbances, nervousness, soreness and weakness in the extremities, symptoms of schizophrenia, walking and speaking difficulties.

Vitamin B15:
Also known as pangamic acid. This substance is not officially recognized as a vitamin, since the official definition of a vitamin states that it must be necessary to health, and there is no sign of deficiency if pangamic acid is not present. However, it is a natural substance which may serve to influence the functions of the body. It is water-soluble, cannot be stored in the body; useful for cell oxidation, respiration; stimulates glucose, fat and protein metabolism; stimulates glandular and nervous system.

Choline:
Water-soluble, cannot be stored in the body. Necessary for the health of the liver, kidney and nervous tissue; helps prevent gallstones; combined with inositol, it is the basic constituent of lecithin for utilization of fats.

Deficiency symptoms include: bleeding ulcers, fatty liver, growth problems, high blood pressure, kidney problems.

Biotin:
Also known as vitamin H. Water-soluble, destroyed by air. Necessary for growth, lipid synthesis in liver, metabolism of carbohydrates, fats and protein; necessary for vitamin B utilization.

Deficiency symptoms include: dry skin, eczema, grayish skin, hair loss, insomnia, irregular heartbeat, mental depression, muscular pain.

Folic Acid:
Water-soluble, destroyed by heat and light. Aids liver performance, appetite, cell reproduction, growth, hydrochloride production for digestion, protein metabolism and red-blood cell formation.

Deficiency symptoms include: anemia, digestive disturbances, graying hair, mental illness, poor growth, inflammation of the tongue.

Inositol:
Water-soluble, cannot be stored in the body. Necessary for brain-cell nutrition, fat metabolism, growth and survival of cells in bone marrow; necessary for the health of eyes, hair, intestines; necessary for lecithin formation in the body, reduces blood cholesterol, protects liver, kidneys and heart.

Deficiency symptoms include: constipation, eczema, eye abnormalities, hair loss, high blood cholesterol.

Para-amino-benzoic acid (also known as PABA):
Water-soluble, cannot be stored in the body, destroyed by air, cooking, canning, pasteurization, insecticides; necessary for blood-cell formation, hair pigment, stimulates the body to make folic acid; necessary for protein metabolism.

Deficiency symptoms include: constipation, depression,

digestive disturbances, gray hair, headache, irritability, nervousness.

Vitamin C:
Also known as ascorbic acid. Water-soluble, destroyed by cooking, oxidation, canning, pasteurization; necessary for blood vessel health, calcium diffusion, good appetite; prevents vitamin oxidation; promotes growth and healing, proper bone and tooth formation; protects the heart; promotes resistance to infection; necessary for red blood cell formation.

Deficiency symptoms include: anemia, bleeding gums, tendency to bruise easily, capillary ruptures, dental caries, headache, impaired adrenal function, lowered resistance to infection, pernicious anemia, scurvy, ulcers.

Vitamin P:
Also known as bioflavonoids. Water-soluble, must be obtained daily; occurs with vitamin C showing similar properties; increases resistance to colds and flu, maintains healthy connective tissue and blood vessel walls, proper absorption of vitamin C, strengthens capillary walls, alters permeability of capillaries.

Deficiency symptoms: the same as vitamin C.

Vitamin D:
Also known as calciferol. Fat-soluble, stable to light, heat and air; can be stored in the body; necessary for the absorption and metabolism of calcium and phosphorus; necessary for proper heart action, clotting, proper gland function, tooth and bone formation, skin respiration.

Deficiency symptoms include: constipation, dental caries, insomnia, lack of stamina, muscular weakness, myopia, nervousness, poor bone development, rickets.

Vitamin E:
Also known as tocopherol, tocopheryl. Fat-soluble, stable to light and heat. Ultraviolet light destroys it; rancid fats reduce the potency; necessary for fertility, lung protection, blood flow to the heart, male potency, pituitary regulation; helps prevent toxemia in pregnancy, retards aging, helps reduce blood cholesterol, protects against oxidation.

Deficiency symptoms include: brittle and falling hair, deficient lactation, gastrointestinal disease, impotence, miscarriage, sterility.

Vitamin K:
Also known as menadione. Fat-soluble; necessary for blood clotting (prevents hemorrhage), vital for normal liver function; vitality and longevity factor.

Deficiency symptoms include: cellular disease, diarrhea, increased clotting time, nosebleeds, miscarriage.

MINERALS

Calcium:
Aids general mineral and vitamin metabolism, bone/tooth formation, clotting, nerve and muscle response; promotes normal behavior and mental alertness, proper heart action, regulation of pH.

Deficiency symptoms include: bone malformation, cramps, heart palpitations, joint pains, impaired growth, insomnia, nervousness, numbness in extremities.

Copper:
Absorbs and carries oxygen as a component of hemoglobin; increases resistance to stress and disease; necessary for health of all cells.

Deficiency symptoms include: breathing difficulties, brittle nails, constipation, iron deficiency anemia.

Iodine:

Aids nutritive process; balances general glandular system; contributes to the color and texture of hair; necessary for energy production, fat metabolism, proper thyroid function, circulation.

Deficiency symptoms include: cretinism, dry hair, goiter, hardening of arteries, heart palpitations, irritability, obesity, slowed mental reactions, sluggish metabolism.

Iron:

Assists hemoglobin and red blood cell formation; necessary for the oxidation of vitamin C, protein metabolism, RNA synthesis, skin and hair pigmentation, synthesis of phospholipids, proper bone formation.

Deficiency symptoms include: anemia, edema, general weakness, impaired respiration, skin sores.

Magnesium:

Aids in elimination of foreign matter; necessary for the formation of albumen; builds cells particularly of nerve tissue; aids in calcium and vitamin C metabolism; is a constituent of muscle and adds strength to bones and teeth; helps regulate blood pH.

Deficiency symptoms include: apprehensiveness, brain and body exhaustion, confusion, disorientation, glandular disturbances, irritability, muscle twitch, poor circulation, poor complexion, tremors.

Phosphorus:

Necessary for bone and tooth formation, kidney function, metabolism of fats, carbohydrates and protein; aids in nerve transmission, nucleoprotein formation; regulates blood pH and skeletal growth.

Deficiency symptoms include: appetite loss, irregular breathing, mental and physical fatigue, nervous disorders, weight irregularity.

Potassium:
Assists kidney function, balances acids, counterbalances sodium action, gives pliancy to muscle tissue; essential to glycogen formation, maintaining proper fluid balance, necessary for normal growth.

Deficiency symptoms include: acne, constipation, dry skin, general weakness, nervous disorders, poor reflexes, thirst, irregular heart beat.

Sodium:
Helps eliminate carbon dioxide; helps form digestive juices, saliva, bile, pancreatic juice, keeps blood minerals soluble, necessary for muscle contraction, regulates water balance and blood pH.

Deficiency symptoms include: appetite loss, gas, impaired fat conversion, muscle shrinkage, vomiting, weight loss.

Sulphur:
Has an antiseptic effect on alimentary tract, is a constituent of hemoglobin, helps keep hair glossy and healthy, complexion clear, maintains body resistance and matures cells, helps to normalize heart action, prevent toxic accumulation, purifies blood and stimulates bile.

Deficiency symptoms include: brittle nails and splitting hair.

Selenium:
Protects against harmful oxidative reactions; protects against harmful effects of cadmium and mercury; works with vitamin E as an antioxidant and protects tissues.

Deficiency symptoms include: premature aging, arteriosclerosis, retarded growth in children.

Chromium:

Necessary for the metabolism of glucose, increases effect of insulin, stimulates synthesis of fatty acids.

Deficiency symptoms include: glucose intolerance, hypoglycemia, diabetes, atherosclerosis.

Zinc:

Necessary for vitamin B1 carbohydrate assimilation, healing of burns and wounds, maintenance of healthy tissue, normal prostate function; needed for phosphorus and protein metabolism; necessary for reproductive organ growth and development.

Deficiency symptoms include: decreased alertness, delayed sexual maturity, fatigue, loss of taste, prolonged healing time, retarded growth, sterility.

HANDY REFERENCE CHART

Greatest concentrations of the following vitamins are found in the indicated fruits and vegetables. That does not mean that other foods do not have the nutrients indicated, but that the quantity may be less.

Vitamins and Enzymes

VITAMIN A	Occurs as pro-vitamin A (carotene) in fruits and vegetables. This is transformed by the body into usable vitamin A. Carrots, green and red peppers, strawberries, oranges and other citrus fruits, parsley, watercress.
VITAMIN B1	Grapefruit, spinach, dandelion.
VITAMIN B2	Parsley, spinach, kale.

VITAMIN B3   Parsley, potatoes, asparagus.

VITAMIN B5   Cabbage, cauliflower, strawberries, grapefruit, oranges.

VITAMIN B6   Pears, spinach, potatoes, lemons, carrots.

FOLIC ACID   Spinach, parsley, potatoes, oranges.

BIOTIN   Cauliflower, spinach, lettuce, grapefruit.

INOSITOL   Oranges, grapefruit, cauliflower, kale, onions.

VITAMIN C   Black currants, citrus fruits, green peppers, nettles, parsley, rosehips.

VITAMIN K   Nettles, spinach, cabbage.

VITAMIN P   Grapes, oranges, currants, rosehips, plums, green peppers.

VITAMIN E   Many cold pressed vegetable oils, wheat germ oil.

ENZYMES   All raw juices. Enzymes are made inactive by heating over 60° centigrade.

Minerals

CALCIUM   Lemons, tangerines, elderberries, nettles, kohlrabi, watercress, turnip tops.

POTASSIUM   Grapes, tangerines, lemons, spinach, kale, potatoes, and most green leafy vegetables.

SODIUM   Elderberries, raspberries, lemons, endive, nettles.

PHOSPHORUS   Grapes, raspberries, tangerines, spinach, watercress, kale.

SULFUR   Black and red currants, spinach, watercress, kale, onion, garlic.

IRON   Red and black currants, raspberries, spinach, apricots, parsley, nettles.

COPPER   Black and red currants, kale, potatoes, asparagus.

MANGANESE   Strawberries, apricots, oranges, lettuce,

spinach, kale.

ZINC	Apples, pears, kale, lettuce, asparagus.
COBALT	Apples; yellow onions.
FLUORINE*	Black currants, cherries, spinach, carrots.
IODINE	Spinach, oranges.
SILICON	Strawberries, grapes, lettuce, carrots.

All of these vitamins and minerals are known to the body. What do you think the body does when confronted with a mess of chemicals disguised as food? You know the products I mean. It can be a product to put into coffee instead of milk or cream, or something that looks like whipped cream—and these are only two examples. The rest are on the supermarket shelf. Look for them if only to avoid problems.

It's not that they don't taste good. They should! Millions of dollars in research money has insured that they will delight your mouth, but what will they do for your cells?

Your body does not know how to handle these strange materials. Spokesmen for the manufacturers will try to convince you that all food is chemical in nature. That's true: all foods and all of us are chemical in nature; but it's the arrangement of the chemicals that make you you, me me and an apple an apple! There's no way any scientist can take an apple, break it down into its chemical parts, put it back together and end up with a pear.

Give your body the raw materials it needs from the foods it knows and trusts.

*This Fluorine is naturally occurring, and, while there is some controversy about the amount needed in human nutrition, there is no question about its place, providing it comes from natural sources.

8. *Juice in Sickness and in Health*

::

THE FOLLOWING AILMENTS and juice formulas* are listed as a guide to the health professional and for general information. They are not intended to be prescriptive. We recommend that all illness be treated by a physician, particularly one who is familiar with alternative healing methods.

ACNE

1. Carrot juice	16 ounces daily
2. Carrot juice	6 ounces
Spinach juice	6 ounces
Lettuce juice	4 ounces
mixture daily	
3. Carrot juice	10 ounces
Spinach juice	6 ounces
mixture daily in divided doses	
4. Asparagus juice	6 ounces daily
if there is a problem of water retention as well.	

*(A number of mixtures will be given for each condition. It is not necessary to use all of the formulas. One 16-ounce mixture a day is sufficient.)

ADDISON'S DISEASE

1. Carrot juice	7 ounces
Lettuce juice	5 ounces

	Pomegranate juice	4 ounces
2.	Celery juice	7 ounces
	Lettuce juice	5 ounces
	Spinach juice	4 ounces

ADENOIDS

In this instance a combination is suggested:

1.	Carrot juice	16 ounces

once a day plus one of the following mixtures

2.	Comfrey juice	10 ounces
	Horseradish (grated)	1 ounce
3.	Onion juice	6 ounces
	Garlic juice	½ ounce
	Horseradish (grated)	1 ounce
4.	Spinach juice	8 ounces
	Dandelion juice	4 ounces
	Comfrey juice	4 ounces

ALLERGY

1.	Carrot juice	10 ounces
	Spinach juice	6 ounces
2.	Carrot juice	8 ounces
	Beet root juice	8 ounces
3.	Carrot juice	8 ounces
	Potato juice	8 ounces
4.	Carrot juice	12 ounces
	Celery juice	4 ounces

ANEMIA

(Simple anemia, not pernicious anemia)

1.	Carrot juice	9 ounces
	Fennel juice	7 ounces
2.	Carrot juice	10 ounces
	Dandelion juice	3 ounces
	Turnip juice	3 ounces

3. Carrot juice   6 ounces
   Fennel juice   6 ounces
   Beetroot juice   4 ounces
4. Watercress juice   2 ounces
   Horseradish (grated)   1 ounce
   Spinach juice   12 ounces
5. Nettle juice   10 ounces
   Watercress juice   2 ounces
   Beetroot juice   4 ounces
6. Turnip-top juice   4 ounces
   Carrot juice   4 ounces
   Spinach juice   4 ounces
   Watercress juice   2 ounces

ANTIBIOTIC THERAPY

Good bacteria as well as bad bacteria are destroyed during therapy. You must restore the gastric flora. Eat some yogurt daily. Drink 16 ounces of any of the following throughout the day.

1. Apple juice   16 ounces
2. Papaya juice   16 ounces
3. Cucumber juice   10 ounces
   Garlic juice   ½ ounce
   Onion juice   2 ounces

ARTERIES

Walk a lot, take vitamin supplements, especially vitamin E. Start with formula No. 1 and take a different formula every day.

1. Carrot juice   10 ounces
   Spinach juice   6 ounces
2. Carrot juice   8 ounces
   Beetroot juice   4 ounces
   Celery juice   4 ounces
3. Carrot juice   8 ounces

Celery juice	4 ounces
Spinach juice	2 ounces
Parsley juice	2 ounces
4. Carrot juice	8 ounces
Nettle juice	8 ounces
5. Pineapple juice	6 ounces
Garlic juice	2 ounces
Carrot juice	8 ounces
6. Pineapple juice	8 ounces
Papaya juice	8 ounces
7. Horseradish (grated)	1 ounce
Garlic juice	2 ounces
Carrot juice	13 ounces
8. Carrot juice	8 ounces
Lettuce juice	4 ounces
Spinach juice	4 ounces

ARTHRITIS

1. Take up to two pints of celery juice daily plus one of the following combinations daily.

2. Spinach	8 ounces
Parsley	2 ounces
Cucumber, or Nettle juice	6 ounces
3. Grapefruit juice	16 ounces
4. Carrot juice	10 ounces
Spinach juice	6 ounces
5. Carrot juice	10 ounces
Beetroot juice	3 ounces
Cucumber juice	3 ounces

ASTHMA

Try a number of different combinations of juices to see which combination is best for you. Avoid concentrated carbohydrates and any food that is mucus-forming.

1. Carrot juice	11 ounces

	Radish juice	5 ounces
2.	Carrot juice	10 ounces
	Celery juice	6 ounces
3.	Carrot juice	5 ounces
	Watercress juice	5 ounces
	Parsley juice	2 ounces
	Potato juice	4 ounces
4.	Horseradish grated	4 ounces
	Lemon juice	4 ounces
	Water	12 ounces
5.	Grapefruit juice	16 ounces

BILIOUSNESS

The failure of the body to produce enough bile to digest fats. Discontinue eating fried foods and stop drinking alcoholic beverages.

1.	Carrot juice	10 ounces
	Celery juice	4 ounces
	Parsley juice	2 ounces
2.	Cucumber juice	4 ounces
	Carrot juice	8 ounces
	Beetroot juice	4 ounces
3.	Dandelion juice	8 ounces
	Watercress juice	2 ounces
	Nettle juice	4 ounces
4.	Carrot juice	10 ounces
	Spinach juice	6 ounces

BLADDER TROUBLES

1.	Carrot juice	10 ounces
	Beet juice	3 ounces
	Cucumber juice	3 ounces
2.	Carrot juice	10 ounces
	Spinach juice	6 ounces
3.	Cranberry juice	16 ounces

BONES AND TEETH

For young and old there is a continuing need for calcium. Take a pint a day of any combination of the following:

Beetroot leaves	Kale
Cabbage	Leeks
Celery	Parsley
Chard	Turnip tops
Dandelion	Watercress

BRONCHITIS

If it is due to smoking, stop smoking! If the inflammation is due to excess mucus in the bronchial tubes, try the following:

1. Horseradish, grated   4 ounces
   Lemon juice   2 ounces
   Water   12 ounces
2. Turnip juice   10 ounces
   Lemon juice   4 ounces
   Water   2 ounces
3. Cabbage juice   14 ounces
   Garlic juice   2 ounces
4. To cut mucus from the throat area:
   Pineapple juice   8 ounces
5. To restore strength:
   Carrot juice   10 ounces
   Beetroot juice   5 ounces
   Cucumber juice   1 ounce

CHRONIC CATARRH

May be due to cigarettes, or inability to digest milk or starches, or possibly an overweight condition.

1. Horseradish, grated   4 ounces
   Lemon juice   2 ounces
   Water   12 ounces
2. Papaya juice   8 ounces

	Pineapple juice	4 ounces
	Grapefruit juice	4 ounces
3.	Carrot juice	10 ounces
	Radish juice	4 ounces
	Parsley juice	2 ounces

CIRCULATION

Exercise, and take vitamins

1.	Horseradish, grated	3 ounces
	Carrot juice	13 ounces

COLDS

Vitamin C, vitamin A, bee propolis, hot lemon juice

1.	Carrot juice	12 ounces
	Radish juice	4 ounces
2.	Carrot juice	7 ounces
	Celery juice	6 ounces
	Radish juice	3 ounces
3.	Carrot juice	9 ounces
	Beet juice	3 ounces
	Cucumber juice	4 ounces
4.	Carrot juice	10 ounces
	Spinach juice	6 ounces

COLIC

1.	Carrot juice	10 ounces
	Spinach juice	6 ounces
2.	Carrot juice	10 ounces
	Beet juice	3 ounces
	Cucumber juice	3 ounces

Not all gas pains in the abdominal region are due to the retention of food wastes in the system or to improper food combining (such as protein plus concentrated carbohydrates). If you suspect a cause other than stated, please call your doctor.

COLITIS

Eat more unprocessed bran or bran cereal. Drink the juice of a lemon in a glass of hot water first thing on arising.

1. Apple juice   10 ounces
   Carrot juice   6 ounces
2. Beetroot juice   8 ounces
   Carrot juice   4 ounces
   Cucumber juice   4 ounces
3. Papaya juice   16 ounces
4. Carrot juice   10 ounces
   Spinach juice   6 ounces

CONSTIPATION

Add unprocessed bran to your diet. Eat yogurt daily. Try some blackstrap molasses mixed with the yogurt.

1. Carrot juice   10 ounces
   Spinach juice   6 ounces
2. Carrot juice   8 ounces
   Apple juice   8 ounces
3. Potato juice   16 ounces
4. Carrot juice   9 ounces
   Beet juice   4 ounces
   Cucumber juice   3 ounces

CONVALESCENCE

All juices are helpful, as are exercise and fresh air. Try fennel, string beans, beetroot, carrot or parsley.

DERMATITIS

Try applying some aloe vera juice directly to the irritation. Or some avocado pulp or papaya juice and pulp, or some yogurt.

1. Carrot juice   6 ounces
   Apple juice   6 ounces

	Celery juice	4 ounces
2.	Carrot juice	8 ounces
	Celery juice	8 ounces
3.	Carrot juice	10 ounces
	Parsley juice	2 ounces
	Watercress juice	4 ounces

DIABETES

Must be treated by a physician. Helpful juices include:

1.	Brussels sprout juice	8 ounces
	String bean juice	8 ounces
2.	Carrot juice	6 ounces
	Lettuce juice	4 ounces
	String bean juice	3 ounces
	Brussels sprout juices	3 ounces
3.	Lemon juice	2 ounces
	Horseradish, grated	2 ounces
	Water	12 ounces
4.	Carrot juice	9 ounces
	Celery juice	5 ounces
	Parsley juice	2 ounces

DIARRHEA

Persistent cases require a physician. If natural cleansing is called for, some of these will help.

1.	Carrot juice	7 ounces
	Celery juice	4 ounces
	Parsley juice	2 ounces
	Spinach juice	3 ounces
2.	Beetroot juice	8 ounces
	Cabbage juice	8 ounces
3.	Beetroot juice	8 ounces
	Garlic juice	2 ounces
4.	Cabbage juice	6 ounces
	Garlic juice	1 ounce

	Nettle juice	7 ounces
5.	Papaya juice	8 ounces
	Pineapple juice	8 ounces

DYSENTERY

Treat as above, but replace the lost fluid by drinking at least four pints of any of the above or plain water.

DYSPEPSIA

See under *indigestion*

ECZEMA

Should be treated by a physician. Many causes, possibly hereditary. Often brought on by stress, sometimes due to diet or alcohol. Try a vegetarian diet for a while to see if it clears the condition.

1.	Spinach juice	5 ounces
	Carrot juice	11 ounces
2.	Potato juice	10 ounces
3.	Carrot juice	9 ounces
	Beet juice	3 ounces
	Lettuce juice (green leaves only)	4 ounces
4.	Carrot juice	7 ounces
	Celery juice	4 ounces
	Parsley juice	2 ounces
	Spinach juice	3 ounces
5.	Papaya juice	12 ounces
6.	Nettle juice	4 ounces
	Carrot juice	10 ounces
	Lettuce juice	2 ounces

EMPHYSEMA

Must be treated by a physician. Some patients report they have been helped by juice in conjunction with medical treatment.

1. Watercress juice 2 ounces
   Potato juice 4 ounces
   Carrot juice 7 ounces
   Parsnip juice 3 ounces
2. Watercress juice 6 ounces
3. Potato juice 6 ounces

ENURESIS

1. Carrot juice 10 ounces
   Beetroot juice 3 ounces
   Cucumber juice 3 ounces
2. Carrot juice 10 ounces
   Celery juice 4 ounces
   Parsley juice 2 ounces
3. Carrot juice 10 ounces
   Beetroot juice 3 ounces
   Coconut juice 3 ounces

EYES

All eye troubles should be dealt with by a physician. In cases of night-blindness brought about by a lack of vitamin A, the following will be useful.

1. Carrot juice 10 ounces
   Fennel juice 6 ounces
2. Carrot juice 12 ounces
   Parsley juice 1 ounce
   Watercress juice 2 ounces
3. Carrot juice 8 ounces
   Celery juice 8 ounces
4. Carrot juice 8 ounces
   Fennel juice 4 ounces
5. Papaya juice 16 ounces
6. Carrot juice 8 ounces
   Spinach juice 2 ounces

Celery juice   6 ounces

FATIGUE

If it is chronic, it can be an indication that the cells of the body are not getting the energy they need from the food you are eating. It is also possible that fatigue can be the precursor of a disease. Try rest, fresh air and plenty of raw juices. If the condition does not improve, see a physician.

1. Grapefruit juice   16 ounces
2. Orange juice   16 ounces
3. Grapefruit juice   8 ounces
   Lemon juice   2 ounces
   Orange juice   6 ounces
4. Carrot juice   16 ounces
5. Spinach juice   6 ounces
   Carrot juice   10 ounces
6. Beetroot juice   3 ounces
   Cucumber juice   3 ounces
   Carrot juice   10 ounces
7. Orange juice   8 ounces
   Apple juice   6 ounces
   Lettuce juice   1 ounce
   Lemon juice   1 ounce

FEVER

Is not the bad thing most people think. It is the body's effort to burn out something that it wants to get rid of. Drink all the juices you can: citrus, celery, grape.

1. Cabbage juice   10 ounces
   Onion juice   1 ounce
   Garlic juice   1 ounce

FRACTURES

To heal a broken bone, the body requires calcium and

silicon as well as vitamin C and all the other nutrients.

1.	Comfrey juice	16 ounces
2.	Carrot juice	8 ounces
	Milk	8 ounces
3.	Carrot juice	8 ounces
	Comfrey juice	8 ounces

Also take silica tablets, available in your health food store.

GALLSTONES

Require treatment by a physician. Avoid fatty foods, lose weight!

1.	Apple juice	10 ounces
	Celery juice	6 ounces
2.	Carrot juice	10 ounces
	Beetroot juice	3 ounces
	Coconut juice	3 ounces
3.	Carrot juice	10 ounces
	Cucumber juice	3 ounces
	Beetroot juice	3 ounces
4.	Carrot juice	10 ounces
	Spinach juice	6 ounces
5.	Nettle juice	4 ounces
	Watercress juice	4 ounces
	Carrot juice	8 ounces
6.	Celery juice	16 ounces

GOITER

Should be treated by a physician. Usually caused by too little iodine in the diet. Add organic iodine to the diet with kelp, dulse or sea lettuce.

1.	Parsley juice	1 ounce
	Carrot juice	8 ounces
	Celery juice	7 ounces
2.	Carrot juice	6 ounces

	Celery juice	4 ounces
	Spinach juice	4 ounces
	Parsley juice	2 ounces
3.	Carrot juice	10 ounces
	Spinach juice	6 ounces
4.	Carrot juice	10 ounces
	Spinach juice	4 ounces
	Watercress juice	2 ounces

GOUT

You can have an ounce or so of whiskey but no wine or beer. No anchovies, no sardines. Try a vegetarian diet for a month to see the results. At any rate, reduce all fats in the diet to zero for a while.

1.	String bean juice	6 ounces
	Drink this every day.	
2.	Carrot juice	10 ounces
	Celery juice	4 ounces
	Parsley juice	2 ounces
3.	Carrot juice	6 ounces
	Spinach juice	6 ounces

HEMORRHOIDS

Add unprocessed bran to your diet and see your doctor. Helpful juices include:

1.	Potato juice	8 ounces
	Watercress juice	8 ounces
2.	Carrot juice	10 ounces
	Spinach juice	6 ounces
3.	Turnip juice	2 ounces
	Watercress juice	2 ounces
	Carrot juice	12 ounces
4.	Nettle juice	1 ounce after meals and at bedtime.

HAIR LOSS

Usually it's a condition you can blame on your father and mother for not choosing parents who didn't go bald. Try nettle juice internally and rub a little on your head at the same time. It can't hurt!

1. Alfalfa juice — 6 ounces
   Lettuce juice — 4 ounces
   Carrot juice — 6 ounces
2. Spinach juice — 8 ounces
   Lettuce juice — 8 ounces

HAY FEVER

If it's the area you live in, move when the sneezes attack. The best cure is to avoid the substance that causes the outbreak. Failing that, try some of these juices.

1. Celery juice — 8 ounces
   Carrot juice — 6 ounces
2. Beetroot juice — 6 ounces
   Cucumber juice — 4 ounces
   Carrot juice — 6 ounces
3. Horseradish, grated — 2 ounces
   Lemon juice — 1 ounce
   Water — 12 ounces
4. Carrot juice — 6 ounces
   Celery juice — 6 ounces
   Spinach juice — 2 ounces
   Parsley juice — 2 ounces

HEADACHE

If headaches are persistent, it is best to consult a physician. If they are a result of diet, they may be prevented by a change of diet from refined foods to raw vegetables and increased grains. Add a cereal that's rich in unprocessed bran.

1. Apple juice   8 ounces
   Parsley juice   2 ounces
   Tomato juice   6 ounces
2. Cabbage juice   12 ounces
   Celery juice   4 ounces
3. Carrot juice   8 ounces
   Beetroot juice   4 ounces
   Cucumber juice   4 ounces
4. Cabbage juice   10 ounces
   Beetroot juice   6 ounces

INDIGESTION

If chronic, see your physician. Can come from improper food combining, or not enough acid in the stomach. There are two acid conditions in the stomach: one is hydrochloric acid that is necessary for the digestion of food, and the other is putrefactive acid that is the result of incomplete digestion. Frequently it is a lack of hydrochloric acid that leads to what is called, erroneously, an acid condition. Try different juices to see if you can find one that will help your condition.

1. Cabbage juice   16 ounces
2. Papaya juice   16 ounces
3. Carrot juice   10 ounces
   Beetroot juice   3 ounces
   Cucumber juice   3 ounces
4. Carrot juice   10 ounces
   Spinach juice   6 ounces
5. Pineapple juice   16 ounces
6. Tomato juice   16 ounces
7. Carrot juice   7 ounces
   Beetroot juice   6 ounces
   Lettuce juice   3 ounces

INFLUENZA

Call in a physician. Prevention is the best medicine. Winter can be hazardous to your health unless you build up your resistance all year long. Older people in particular should take vitamin supplements all year.

1. Carrot juice — 6 ounces
   Potato juice — 6 ounces
   Parsley juice — 2 ounces
   Watercress — 2 ounces
2. Carrot juice — 8 ounces
   Celery juice — 8 ounces
3. Carrot juice — 7 ounces
   Parsley juice — 2 ounces
   Spinach juice — 3 ounces
   Celery juice — 4 ounces
4. Carrot juice — 8 ounces
   Celery juice — 5 ounces
   Radish juice — 3 ounces

KIDNEYS

Need sufficient fluid every day. Water is important and so is juice, particularly the following:

1. Celery juice — 6 ounces
   Beetroot juice — 6 ounces
   Cucumber juice — 4 ounces
2. Carrot juice — 8 ounces
   Beetroot juice — 4 ounces
   Celery juice — 4 ounces
3. Dandelion juice — 2 ounces
   Watercress juice — 2 ounces
   Lettuce juice — 4 ounces
   Carrot juice — 8 ounces

LARYNGITIS

Don't strain to talk. It's important not to put extra

stress on the larynx. Take some lemon juice in water and use it as a gargle. Sip some honey. Chew on a mixture of onion, garlic and apple-cider vinegar.

1. Pineapple juice   8 ounces
   Carrot juice   8 ounces
2. Pineapple juice   16 ounces
3. Carrot juice   10 ounces
   Spinach juice   6 ounces
4. Carrot juice   10 ounces
   Cucumber juice   3 ounces
   Beetroot juice   3 ounces
5. Apple juice   8 ounces
   Carrot juice   8 ounces

LIVER PROBLEMS

Can be caused by too much alcohol, wine or beer, or a diet of highly concentrated sugar, starch, fats and meat and not enough raw vegetables and fruit. Also, the B-complex vitamins may be in short supply. Use supplements and drink juice.

1. Apple juice   16 ounces
2. Carrot juice   8 ounces
   Celery juice   8 ounces
3. Carrot juice   10 ounces
   Beetroot juice   4 ounces
   Coconut juice   2 ounces
4. Asparagus juice   4 ounces
   Dandelion juice   4 ounces

LOW BLOOD PRESSURE

See a physician if it's very low and you get dizzy. You need more vital foods in your diet.

1. Carrot juice   10 ounces
   Spinach juice   6 ounces
2. Spinach juice   6 ounces

	Beetroot juice	10 ounces
3.	Carrot juice	5 ounces
	Celery juice	5 ounces
	Watercress juice	2 ounces
	Parsley juice	2 ounces
	Spinach juice	2 ounces

MENSTRUATION, EXCESSIVE

Iron is needed. Organic iron is the best choice. Try a supplement of organic iron, vitamin C, vitamin A, vitamin D, and copper.

1.	Fennel juice	8 ounces
	Beet juice	8 ounces
2.	Carrot juice	6 ounces
	Celery juice	4 ounces
	Spinach juice	4 ounces
	Parsley juice	2 ounces
3.	Beetroot juice	8 ounces
	Nettle juice	8 ounces
4.	Carrot juice	10 ounces
	Fennel juice	6 ounces
5.	Cabbage juice	8 ounces
	Lettuce juice	8 ounces

MENSTRUATION, IRREGULAR

1.	Parsley juice	6 ounces
2.	Fennel juice	6 ounces
	Fig juice	6 ounces
	Parsley juice	4 ounces

MENOPAUSE

A shifting of body gears for easier living.

1.	Carrot juice	8 ounces
	Beetroot juice	4 ounces
	Pomegranate juice	4 ounces

2.	Carrot juice	8 ounces
	Spinach juice	8 ounces
3.	Parsley juice	2 ounces
	Celery juice	4 ounces
	Carrot juice	7 ounces
	Spinach juice	3 ounces
4.	Carrot juice	6 ounces
	Turnip juice	3 ounces
	Beetroot juice	3 ounces
	Lettuce juice	4 ounces

MUCOUS MEMBRANE (DRY)

Supplement with vitamin A, zinc gluconate, vitamin B2.

1.	Carrot juice	8 ounces
	Celery juice	8 ounces
2.	Carrot juice	8 ounces
	Pineapple juice	4 ounces
	Papaya juice	4 ounces
3.	Carrot juice	5 ounces
	Beetroot juice	5 ounces
	Cucumber juice	5 ounces
	Lemon juice	1 ounce

NERVOUSNESS

Can be caused by organic alkaline shortage, and many other problems. If it is caused by a dietary deficiency, try these:

1.	Dandelion juice	6 ounces
	Nettle juice	6 ounces
2.	Brussels sprout juice	4 ounces
	String bean juice	6 ounces
3.	Carrot juice	10 ounces
	Beetroot juice	3 ounces
	Cucumber juice	3 ounces

    4. Carrot juice   10 ounces
       Celery juice with tops   6 ounces

PEPTIC; DUODENAL; AND GASTRIC ULCERS
See your physician! And try:
    1. Cabbage juice   16 ounces
    2. Cabbage juice   8 ounces
       Carrot juice   8 ounces
    3. Pineapple juice   8 ounces
       Papaya juice   8 ounces
    4. Comfrey juice   12 ounces
    5. Potato juice   16 ounces

PROSTATE TROUBLE
Some nutritionists recommend zinc gluconate and pumpkin seed oil. See your physician.
    1. Lettuce juice   5 ounces
       Asparagus juice   5 ounces
       Carrot juice   6 ounces
    2. Beetroot juice   16 ounces
    3. Carrot juice   8 ounces
       Beet juice   4 ounces
       Cucumber juice   4 ounces
    4. Spinach juice   8 ounces
       Carrot juice   8 ounces

RHEUMATISM
Build strength and wash out waste material.
    1. Beetroot juice   8 ounces
       Watercress juice   4 ounces
       Cucumber juice   4 ounces
    2. Celery juice   5 ounces
       Cucumber juice   5 ounces
       Carrot juice   11 ounces
    3. Celery juice   8 ounces

Carrot juice	8 ounces
4. Spinach juice	6 ounces
Carrot juice	10 ounces
5. Cherry juice	16 ounces

SEXUAL DRIVE, WEAKENED

Nutritionists recommend vitamin E, honey and bee pollen. Herbalists like damiana, dong qui, and ginseng tea. Try everything!

1. Beetroot juice	16 ounces
2. Celery juice	16 ounces
3. Carrot juice	8 ounces
Beetroot juice	4 ounces
Cucumber juice	4 ounces

SINUS TROUBLE

1. Lemon juice	2 ounces
Horseradish, grated	1 ounce
Water	12 ounces
2. Carrot juice	8 ounces
Radish juice with leaves	4 ounces
Pineapple juice	4 ounces
3. Carrot juice	8 ounces
Papaya juice	8 ounces
4. Radish juice	2 ounces
Garlic juice	1 ounce
Onion juice	1 ounce
Lemon juice	1 ounce
Water	11 ounces

SKIN BLEMISHES

Vitamin A, zinc gluconate, pH balanced soap, balanced diet.

1. Apple juice	12 ounces
2. Beetroot juice	12 ounces

3.	Cabbage juice	6 ounces
	Carrot juice	10 ounces
4.	Potato juice	10 ounces
	Quince juice	2 ounces
	Cucumber juice	2 ounces
	Carrot juice	2 ounces
5.	Asparagus juice	8 ounces
	Dandelion juice	4 ounces
	Watercress juice	2 ounces
	Carrot juice	2 ounces

VARICOSITY (CAUSED BY CONSTIPATION)

Add bran to your diet. Eat whole grains. Eat one container of yogurt daily.

1.	Apple juice	12 ounces
2.	Asparagus juice	2 ounces
	Potato juice	12 ounces
3.	Carrot juice	8 ounces
	Spinach juice	4 ounces
	Turnip juice	2 ounces
	Watercress juice	2 ounces

WATER RETENTION

There are many causes, and you should see your physician. Juices with diuretic properties can be useful.

1.	Asparagus juice	6 ounces
2.	Celery juice	16 ounces
3.	Dandelion juice	12 ounces
4.	Nettle juice	6 ounces
5.	Cucumber juice	8 ounces
	Celery juice	8 ounces
6.	Dandelion juice	8 ounces
	Asparagus juice	4 ounces

WOUNDS (to help the healing process)

Zinc gluconate, vitamins C and K, good protein sources.

1. Alfalfa juice   6 ounces
    Comfrey juice   6 ounces
    Carrot juice   4 ounces

9. *A Cleansing Fast (with Juices)*

IT IS the opinion of most nutritionists that the average person can fast safely, without supervision, for from one to three days. Any fast longer than three days should not be undertaken without medical guidance.

I am in favor of one- to- three-day juice fast, but I do not like a fast that offers water only. Also, a fast that lasts longer than three days can have many side effects. Many toxic substances are stored in fatty tissue where they do the least amount of harm. A long fast will break down the fatty tissue, releasing the toxins into the system. The system can get overloaded and not be able to get rid of the waste material fast enough. The result is not pleasant. The faster cannot stray too far away from the bathroom; headaches are common; and no amount of toothpaste and mouthwash will cover up the breath. Fasters have been known to out-camel a camel in a bad-breath duel.

Ah! But a one-day fast will let your body relax a bit from its daily chores. The juice is easily absorbed into the circulatory system and its nutrients are readily transferred into the cells.

Almost everybody can fast, but there are some exceptions. The following conditions do not lend themselves to a fast of any kind. If you suffer from any one of them, never, *never* go on a fast. Pregnant women have been known to fast, but I advise against it because the baby needs a full complement of nutrients every day and it's impossible to predict the outcome.

People should never fast if any of these conditions are known or suspected:

> Tumors
> Bleeding ulcers
> Cancer
> Cerebral disease
> Kidney disease
> Gout
> Liver disease
> Blood disease
> Recent heart trouble
> Active lung disease
> Diabetes
> Senior citizens without the advice of
> their physician

But if you are fairly healthy and want to change your eating habits from the junk-food regime to a more natural food regime, a one-day juice fast to help detoxify your system can be a good start.

If your physician approves, juice fasting can aid a patient in his recovery from certain disease states, since raw juice from fruits and vegetables contains the vitamins, minerals, trace elements and enzymes to speed up the healing process.

You can prepare for your fast by planning a menu of raw fruits and vegetables. At one meal eat only fruit. The next meal should be only vegetables, and so on. Do not mix the fruit and vegetables together. Drink herb tea such as chamomile or peppermint tea flavored with a bit of honey. Do this for two days. Then, you're ready to begin your juice fast.

> Wake up with a smile:

At 7:30 A.M.	Take the juice of a lemon, mix it with 8 ounces of water and drink.
8:30	Take a glass of fresh orange juice.
9:30	Take a glass of tomato juice.
10:30	Make some alfalfa tea and sip it.
11:30	Fresh apple juice—one glass.
12:30	Another 8 ounces of water.
1:30	A glass of grape juice.
	Rest period—nothing at all.
4:30	Pineapple juice.
5:30	Prune juice.
6:30	Peppermint tea, sip slowly.
7:30	Grapefruit juice.
8:30	Chamomile tea.

> Go to bed!

Briefly, here's the rundown on a few of the nutritional values in this simple one-day juice fast.

Protein	9 grams
Calcium	195 mg
Vitamin A	2,620 I.U.
Vitamin C	365 mg
B-complex	35 mg

You'll notice that the juices supply the water-soluble vitamins, the ones we must get daily to help us fight pollution and handle stress problems. They also supply protein for body defense and calcium to make sure of the blood-calcium level. So a juice fast is not a starvation diet!

The key to successful juice fasting is to drink a variety

of fruit juices rather than just one type. In that way you insure a supply of needed nutrients. If you wish to continue the juice fast for two or three days, don't go right into heavy foods on the day after you conclude the fast. The morning after the fast, eat a whole apple or a banana for breakfast. Try some vegetable soup with one slice of seven-grain bread for lunch. Stay on the juices for the rest of the day. The next day, add some mashed potatoes and boiled eggs to your menu. After that add some raw vegetable salad, some boiled rice and some cottage cheese.

If you step on the scale you'll find you've lost some weight but that's only a little bonus. You've detoxified your body and you're ready for the new you.

Of course if you go back to potato chips, sugar and refined flour products . . . shame on you!

10. *What's What in Foods and on Labels*

AFTER you've come off your three-day fast and have decided you like the way you feel, you're ready to go shopping to buy the kinds of food that will help you continue feeling good. There's a complete "How to pick fresh fruit" guide later on in this book but there are a lot of other items on the market that you may not know about. Here's an alphabetical listing with some information that will help you familiarize yourself with these items and then decide if they are something you want to put in your stomach.

Acerola
These are Caribbean cherries that are very rich in vitamin C.

Additives
Don't confuse them with supplements. Additives are usually chemical substances, preservatives, emulsifiers, etc., that are put into products to promote shelf life. No one can honestly say that they are completely safe. Avoid them when you can.

Agar-agar
Comes from the sea. It is a sea vegetable that can be used to thicken sauces the way that starch or gelatin do. It is a good source of sea minerals and vitamins.

Aluminum
Mostly used in pots and pans, aluminum is a soft metal

and can contaminate foods cooked in it. I prefer to use either glass or stainless steel for cooking.

Arrowroot starch
This is a natural thickening agent that can be used instead of white flour, which has lost all of its vitamin and mineral content.

Artificial colorings
These are usually dyes and are potentially toxic. Some manufacturers add them to oranges, lemons, yams and red skinned potatoes. Best to avoid them when you can. Look for natural food colors.

Baking powder
Not the most wanted substance in the world but it's a quick leavener so it's okay to use a little. Try to find the kind without aluminum. Read the label carefully.

Baking soda
This can neutralize stomach acid and prevent proper digestion, so don't put it into cooked food.

BHT and BHA
These two are antioxidants which are added to foods to maintain freshness. They are very popular and found in many products. Although most nutritionists favor banning them. I'm not sure that they are as bad as the other additives. This is one where I'll have to walk the middle line and leave the decision to you.

Barley
Do not buy pearled or polished barley, because you lose a great deal of nutrients with the polishings. Look for the hulled whole grain. Delicious in soups, stews, casseroles or as a substitute for rice or potatoes.

Barley flour
Just what it says, flour ground from barley grain. It

does not contain gluten and will not hold a loaf of bread together, so add it to other flours for baking. Has a good flavor.

Bioflavonoid
Substance found in nature along with vitamin C. It acts with it to protect against allergies, colds, capillary fragility, etc. Usually found under the skin of citrus fruits. Also found in large quantities in buckwheat.

Blackstrap molasses
Rich in nutrients. Twice the amount of iron as liver. Most of the B-complex vitamins, and twice the calcium found in milk. It has a slightly bitter taste and should never be eaten right off the spoon. Mix it with hot water or stir it into milk.

Brewer's yeast
This is a non-leavening yeast. It is an excellent source of the B-vitamin family and one of the most important supplements you can find. It contains seventeen vitamins, fourteen minerals, and sixteen tissue-building amino acids. Store it away from light and it will last a long time. It goes best with strong-tasting dishes where it can be mixed in and disguised. It has a rather strong taste of its own. Start by using just a bit and gradually build the quantity. The flakes tend to dissolve a bit more easily than the powder although the powder is usually more potent. I usually mix it with peanut butter or some other nut butter. Although the heat will destroy some of the B vitamins, making bread dough with brewer's yeast is perhaps the best way to avoid an unpleasant flavor.

Bulgur or Bulghar
Wheat that has been cooked under pressure, dried, and

with the bran partially removed. It is the staff of life in the Near East. Use it like any other cereal grain.

Buttermilk
The protein precipitate in this fermented milk product is in the form of a fine curd which allows for easier digestion than plain milk.

Caffeine
Much controversy about this. It's found in coffee, tea and most soft drinks. It's a stimulant but not nutritious and does you no good whatever.

Carob
If you're allergic to some of the ingredients in chocolate— many people react to the theobromine, a caffeine-like substance—you might try carob. It is a protein-rich food with natural sugar and a taste that resembles chocolate. Try many different brands until you find the one you like best. It is sold under a number of different names, such as "Honey locust," "St. John's Bread," and "Locust Bean."

Carrageen (see Irish moss)

Cellulose
The bulk that regulates body function. It's found in bran, fruits and vegetables. Buy unprocessed bran for best results.

Cheese
Look for aged natural cheeses made without preservatives or artificial coloring. Processed cheeses are to be avoided. Fresh-churned cheese such as cottage, pot or ricotta are high in protein content and easy to digest. Examine the label carefully to make sure there are no additives, and check the date before you buy.

Chocolate & cocoa

Both of these contain saturated fat and can retard digestion. Many people are allergic to them.

Coconut oil

Although this is a vegetable oil, it is highly saturated, whereas all other vegetable oils are unsaturated. It also has less protein than any of the other nuts. On the other hand, coconut meat is a good natural sweetener for desserts, cereals, cake, etc. So, six of one . . .

Coffee

Big, *big* hassle still going on, particularly in the case of pregnant women. The caffeine can't help you and maybe can hurt. Also, the desire to have a sweet cake with it or some other form of refined sugar is a hard habit to break. Herb tea, anyone?

Cold cuts

Very tempting but full of preservatives, nitrates and nitrites. Maybe once in a while, as long as it's a *long* while.

Corn syrup

A way to add refined sugar to a product without calling it refined sugar. Deceitful, to say the least.

Cornell flour formula

Because the refined flours on the market are so lacking in nutritional value that even the bugs can't live on them, Cornell University came up with this formula.

Before you measure the flour in your bread recipe, put 1 tablespoon soya flour, 1 tablespoon dry milk powder and 1 teaspoon wheat germ in the measuring cup. Then fill the cup with flour.

Date sugar

This is a natural sugar prepared from dates that are

dried and then ground. Good on cereals.

Dolomite
A food supplement mined from natural limestone, and one of the best sources of calcium and magnesium.

Dulse
A product from the sea, it is actually a seaweed rich in minerals, vitamins and trace elements. The dried product can be cut up for fish chowders or seafood casseroles.

Flours
Buy wholegrain flour whenever you can, and store it in the refrigerator or freezer. After opening the bag and using some, press the air out before storing again.

WHEAT FLOUR: high gluten content makes dough elastic.

BARLEY FLOUR: blend with other flours in baking muffins.

BUCKWHEAT FLOUR: excellent pancake flour.

CORN FLOUR: used for breading and waffles.

GLUTEN FLOUR: wholegrain wheat with the starch removed.

MILLET FLOUR: for those who are allergic to wheat and other grains.

PEANUT FLOUR: high protein content.

POTATO FLOUR: can be used for cookies, cake and bread.

RICE FLOUR: ground from whole brown rice. Sometimes used for pancakes and waffles.

RYE FLOUR: mix it with wheat in making rye bread.

SOY FLOUR: good fat with high lecithin content. Use with wheat flour in baking.

Fish protein concentrate: called fish flour, but it is not a true flour. It is a deodorized powder that can be added to soups, stews, casseroles, etc., for extra nourishment. It does not taste like fish.

Honey
Try to find organic honey with the words, "raw,

unfiltered" on the label. The range of honey flavors and colors is extensive. The taste varies according to the plant the bees have visited. You can choose among clover, thyme, sage, orange blossom, tupelo, etc. Most people prefer clover honey. Commercial honey may have been treated with high heat and filtered to remove the pollen. If that's the case, some nutritional benefits may have been removed.

Hot dogs
As American as apple pie, but they contain synthetic colors, artificial flavors, fat, phosphates, binders, sodium nitrite or sodium nitrate and don't do you a lot of good.

Hydrogenated
When a nice, liquid vegetable oil is turned into a thick, solid fat, it has been heated with hydrogen. The unsaturated oil is now saturated and, in my opinion, undesirable. If you want a solid fat, use creamery butter.

Irish moss
This is a seaweed that can be used to thicken desserts. It's used in making blancmange. It is sometimes called carrageen or carrageenen. It is very rich in sea minerals and vitamins.

Kasha
This is buckwheat groats.

Kefir
This is a cultured milk beverage made with kefir grains.

Kelp
More seaweed. Wonderfully rich in minerals and vitamins and a great source of organic iodine. Can also be used as a seasoning to replace salt.

Lecithin
A by-product of soybean oil, a rich source of phospha-

tides. Lecithin has a great part to play in the metabolism of cholesterol and helps regulate the amount of cholesterol in the blood. It can be bought in liquid, tablet, capsule and granular form and used daily as a supplement.

Legumes
A food group that includes seeds, nuts, dried beans, peas and lentils. Although they do not have complete protein content individually, when combined correctly they can supply all the essential amino acids.

Malt
This syrup is generally made from germinated barley. It is less sweet than other natural sweeteners.

Maple sugar
This is maple syrup that has been cooked until it granulates. It looks like light brown sugar.

MSG (monosodium glutamate)
Chemically speaking, it is a salt of glutamic acid. Glutamic acid is an amino acid used by the body, and it is on this basis that the user claims it is a natural product. Well, it isn't, and it can cause allergic reactions with a quickened pulse and headache. Some people report excess perspiration as well, and the collection of symptoms has been labeled the "Chinese Food Syndrome," because there is much MSG used in their dishes. When eating out, you can request that they leave out the salt and your request will be honored. MSG has been removed from a lot of foods on the shelves but there's still a lot around. Read your label carefully. If it's in the product, it has to be listed.

Non-dairy milk product
If it's advertised as containing vegetable fat, look to see

if it contains coconut oil. It is a vegetable fat but the only one that's highy saturated. (See section on oils.) The rest of the product is chemical.

Oils

Most nutritionists favor vegetable oils which contain no preservatives, coloring, additives, etc. Store them in the refrigerator and buy them in small quantities. Remember to take extra vitamin E. It is necessary to keep the oils from oxidizing in the body. In fact, E is generally useful for this purpose.

COCONUT OIL:	A highly saturated oil which should be avoided. It is hard to detect its presence in products because it can be listed under the generic term "vegetable oil."
CORN OIL:	Basic oil useful for cooking, baking and salads.
MINERAL OIL:	Never take this at or near meal times. It blocks the body's use of vitamin A, D and E. If taken on a regular basis it can remove these vitamins from the body. There are many other products that can be used as a laxative.
OLIVE OIL:	Buy the first pressing. It has a delicate, very pleasant flavor. Many people like it with salad.
PEANUT OIL:	It is high in unsaturated fatty acids and one of the better oils for baking and frying.
SAFFLOWER OIL:	The highest of all oils in unsaturated fatty acids and the best for salads and light frying. It has a very light flavor that doesn't intrude.

SESAME OIL: High in unsaturated fatty acids. Another good oil for salads.

SOY OIL: High in unsaturated fatty acids. It is a good oil to use in baking, but not for frying, because it will foam. It has a taste of roasted soybeans, which is not unpleasant, but which may affect the taste you are looking for. If you are baking a delicate-tasting muffin, try peanut or safflower oil.

SUNFLOWER OIL: This is another winner. It is highly digestible and highly unsaturated. Excellent for sautéing and frying. You can't go wrong using this oil.

WHEAT GERM OIL: This oil is an important supplement since it is very rich in vitamin E. Each teaspoon contains 10 International Units of vitamin E. It has a heavy taste and can be concealed only by mixing it with a heavy salad dressing.

Organ meats

Nutritionists feel that people in the United States eat the wrong type of meat. Steaks, chops and so on are muscle meat—lots of protein but not much else. Liver, kidney, heart, brains, and lungs are also protein, but in addition supply vitamins and amino acids not found in other meats. You can try mixing the muscle meat with some organ meat when you make hamburger or meat loaf. Your family will not know the difference and they'll get added benefits.

Peanut butter

Look for the old-fashioned type that uses only peanuts

and doesn't add anything. Many health food stores now grind peanut butter and other nut butters fresh for you. Some brands on the market contain salt and sugar. Avoid them.

Polyunsaturates

There is some confusion over the terms polyunsaturated oil and saturated oil. Strictly speaking, a fat that is saturated is a solid at room temperature and is usually a meat or dairy product. Polyunsaturated fats or oils are liquid at room temperature and are vegetable products (except coconut oil). Saturated fats are cholesterol forming while unsaturated oils are not.

Naturally to every rule there must be exceptions. Coconut oil is highly saturated and fish oil, an animal product, is highly unsaturated.

Pumpkin seeds

They are a very nutritious treat. They are called pepita seeds when they are round instead of flat.

Rice

Use the brown rice since it is unrefined and therefore the protein, B-complex vitamins, calcium, phosphorus, iron and copper are still pretty much intact. Only the outermost husk has been removed, so it takes a bit longer to cook than white rice, but the flavor and nutritional value will be your reward.

Ricotta

This is a soft cheese very similar to cottage cheese but less salty and more creamy. If your local store doesn't stock it, try any Italian neighborhood store. You'll be delighted.

Salad dressings

Make your own. Many commercial dressings contain

preservatives that are not beneficial to health.

Salt-free diet
If you're told you should be on one don't use cold cuts, smoked meats or fish, dried beef, ham, cottage cheese, soy sauce, most canned soup, frozen fish, frozen vegetables, sea salt, kelp and read the labels on anything else you buy. You must do most of your own food preparing.

Soft Drinks
Most contain phosphoric acid which causes calcium to be excreted from the body. The citrus-type drinks can contain brominated oils which do not do you *any* good.

Sorghum
This is a natural sweetener made from a grain that is grown like corn.

Soy sauce
Most contain monosodium glutamate. Look for Tamari and check the label. It should be free from MSG.

Sweeteners, natural
Blackstrap molasses, carob powder, carob syrup, date sugar, honey, malt, maple sugar, maple syrup, molasses, sorghum.

Tahini
A paste made from finely ground sesame seeds. It can be used as a spread, as a butter substitute, in salad dressings, or over vegetables. Mix it with honey to prepare homemade halvah.

Tapioca
A root product made from the cassava plant. Get the whole tapioca, not the pearled.

Vanilla
Buy pure vanilla extract or the bean itself. Do not buy vanillin, which is a synthetic product.

Vegetable seasoning
This is a seasoning made from finely ground and dried vegetables. Read the label carefully, because some companies include salt.

Vinegar
Buy apple-cider vinegar made from whole apples. It contains malic acid instead of the acetic acid found in most commercial products. Read labels on malt, white and wine vinegar if you insist on those products. I use them only for cleaning windows.

Whey
The watery part of milk that is separated from the thicker part called the curd when making cheese. Little Miss Muffet sat on a tuffet, having a very nutritious snack.

Yogurt
A calcium-rich, easily digested, cultured milk product. Eat it plain, with nuts or chopped vegetables, as a substitute for sour cream, as a dessert topping or any time.

11. *Juiced for Fun*

NOT EVERYTHING has to be serious.

Nobody likes a bore.

If it can't be fun once in a while, why bother?

This is the part of the book where the juicer's cousin, the blender, comes into its own.

We're going to make beverages that taste good, are fun to drink, can be served at parties, will entice children and even husbands, and can be healthful at the same time.

The only rule is that, wherever possible, the juice must be made fresh. If not possible, use frozen juice as a first choice, and canned juice without added sugar or syrup as a last choice.

Strawberry Shaky
1 cup fresh strawberries
1 cup fresh orange juice
1 tablespoon honey

Blend well and serve over an ice cube. (Delicious—and look at all that vitamin C!)

Yogurt-Tomato Mix
If the kids won't drink tomato juice, let them try this. After you taste it, maybe you won't share it with them!

  2 cups tomato juice
  1 tablespoon yogurt
  ½ teaspoon lemon juice
  ¼ teaspoon white horseradish (or a little less to
  taste)
  ¼ teaspoon of honey (or a little less to taste)
  A dash of sea salt

Blend well and serve over an ice cube.

(Canned tomato juice is one of the few juices that retains its vitamin content—but make sure it does not contain added salt.)

Pineapple-Carrot Surprise

Usually I do not recommend mixing vegetables and fruit because the interaction and the difference in digestive juices can cause gas. However, acid fruits can be mixed with vegetables as in this mixture.

  2 cups pineapple juice
  Juice from 2 carrots
  1 ounce lemon juice

Blend well and serve

Cranberry-Grapefruit Mix

This drink requires a bit of work. You have to wash the cranberries in hot water and then pick out those that don't look good. Peel the grapefruit and scrape off some of the white stuff to add in the juicer.

  Juice of one grapefruit
  Juice of ½ cup of cranberries
  1½ cups water
  2 tablespoons of honey

Blend well.

Not only is this a delicious drink, but it also acts as a diuretic.

Mulled Apple Juice

Have you ever tasted mulled apple juice? It warms you up on a winter's day.

Make 2 quarts of fresh apple juice
Put into a pot and add:
1 inch stick of cinnamon
¼ teaspoon nutmeg
¼ teaspoon allspice
6 whole cloves
⅓ cup of honey

Simmer slowly for twenty minutes and serve in mugs garnished with slices of fresh orange. Wait for the applause!

Mystery Drink

Make them guess what's in it.

Juice 8 large carrots
2 large cucumbers
Add to 8 ounces of coconut juice

Blend well, serve at once.

Pick-me-up

Juice one papaya
one orange
plus the juice of one carrot
blend with ½ cup of yogurt
Add ½ cup more of orange juice and some ice.

Blend at high speed and drink.

Carrot-Apple Drink

Take 1½ cups of fresh carrot juice
½ cup fresh apple juice
1 teaspoon of honey
Dash of cloves

Blend well until it forms a froth.

Orange Nectar

Take ½ cup fresh orange juice and put it in
the blender with 2 soft bananas
3 tablespoons of honey
¼ teaspoon of almond extract
1 quart of milk

Blend until frothy and serve at once.

Watermelon-ade

Puree 2 cups of ripe watermelon
Put it into the blender with
½ cup fresh lemon juice
½ teaspoon grated lemon rind
1 tablespoon of honey
2 cups of water

Blend just until the honey is dissolved.

Summer pick-up

½ cup fresh orange juice
½ cup apple juice
1 teaspoon of lime juice

Stir in a tall glass over ice.

Canteloupe Milk Shake

Throw ½ cup of milk
2 tablespoons of lemon juice
One tablespoon of honey
Cantaloupe meat from a ripe melon

Blend till frothy, serve over ice.

Banana Flip

1 large banana, drawn and quartered
1 tablespoon of honey
⅛ teaspoon of almond extract
A little grated orange rind
1½ cups of cold milk

Blend at high speed. Chill or serve over ice.

Honey/Fruit Punch

Take 1 cup of orange juice
½ cup of lemon juice
½ cup of pineapple juice
2 cups of water
2 teaspoons of honey

Mix, chill, serve cold.

Almost any combination will find favor. You'll have to try a number of combinations for yourself. I'll give you a few more just to keep you tempted.

Fool's Gold

Tastes a lot better than it reads:

> Juice 1 beetroot and
> 5 leaves of romaine lettuce
> and ½ an orange
> and 3 carrots

Blend quickly and drink.

Summer Freshener

> Pineapple juice, about 4 ounces
> Orange juice, about two ounces
> Papaya juice, one ounce
> Carrot juice, one ounce
> Few drops of lime juice

Put in a tall glass and stir.

Celebration Drink

> Chill all the ingredients. Then mix them in a
> mixing bowl, except for the cream.
> 1 pint cream
> ½ cup milk
> ½ cup sweet apple cider
> ½ teaspoonful vanilla extract
> 1 tablespoon of honey, a pinch of nutmeg and
> a tablespoon of sherry

After they're all mixed, beat the cream lightly and add to the mixture. Serve at once and watch all the smiles come out. Have some yourself, but don't make it a habit. It's okay to bend the rules once in a while.

South Sea Delight

Put all of these in the blender:

    2 tablespoons of honey
    1 small apple, unpeeled, quartered and cored
    ½ cup fresh orange or grapefruit juice
    1 cup fresh papaya
    2 teaspoons of peanut butter (that's right, *peanut*)

Blend for about one minute and serve.

Pear Cooler

When pears are in season:
Core two fresh pears and cut in half. Then dice and place them in the blender.
Add the juice from three apricots and:

    ¼ cup lemon juice
    1 tablespoon honey
    ½ cup crushed ice

Blend until smooth.

Thirst Quencher

    1 cup fresh apple juice
    1 cup orange juice
    ½ carrot, sliced
    1 rib of celery
    ½ banana
    2 green leaves of romaine lettuce or spinach
    1 teaspoon of crushed almonds
    1 teaspoon of raisins
    2 sprigs of parsley

Blend well until liquified, then add a bit of crushed ice and blend a few seconds more.

Sexy Vegetable Juice

In the blender:

> 2 tomatoes
> 1 pepper
> 1 carrot and its top
> 2 onions
> 1 cabbage leaf, green

Blend for about two minutes.

Hot Cider Punch

> ½ gallon fresh cider
> 3 cups fresh pineapple juice
> 1½ cups fresh orange juice
> 1 cup honey
> 1 cup lemon juice
> 4 cloves
> 1 stick of cinnamon

Put everything in a kettle. Gently warm and stir until the honey dissolves. Strain into glasses. Makes about 3½ quarts.

Apple Swinger

> ¾ cup fresh apple juice
> ¼ cup celery leaves
> 2 teaspoons lemon juice
> ½ cup cracked ice

Blend and put into two glasses.

Breakfast on the Run

In the blender:

> 2 tablespoons of soya powder
> 1 banana, mashed
> 1 tablespoon honey
> ½ teaspoon vanilla
> 1 pint of cold water

Blend well. Serves two.

Vitamin Gold Mine

In the blender:

> 3 tablespoons carob powder
> 1 level teaspoon brewer's yeast
> 2 teaspoons of honey
> ⅓ cup dry skim milk powder
> ¾ cup water
> two ice cubes

Blend at low speed.

Thick Shake

In the blender:

> 1 cup skim milk
> ½ cup any fruit juice
> ½ teaspoon vanilla extract
> 3 ice cubes

Blend into a frothy drink.

Waist-Watcher

In the blender:

> ¾ cup cold skim milk
> ½ cup blueberries
> 1 teaspoon vanilla

Blend well. If you want it cold, add an ice cube.

Milk of the Lion

In the blender:

> 2 tablespoons dry milk powder
> ½ cup liquid skim milk
> 1 tablespoon tahini paste
> 1 tablespoon blackstrap molasses
> 2 tablespoons of any soft nut
> ½ cup of any fresh fruit

Blend until foamy, then drink.

Romeo and Orange Juliet

In the blender:

> 1 cup fresh orange juice
> ¼ cup dried milk
> 1 tablespoon honey
> 2 drops vanilla extract
> 2 ice cubes

Blend well.

12. *Please Squeeze the Fruit*

ALL through this book I've stressed the use of fruit and vegetables and the nutrients they contain. That presupposes we can pick and get fresh, ripe fruit. It also presupposes that we know how to separate good fruit from bad fruit.

I am a child of the Depression and I remember following my grandmother as she walked through the markets. I had the job of carrying home what she bought. That little old lady was the terror of the markets. No amount of—"Please' lady, *don't* squeeze the fruit!"—could stop her from touching, smelling, prodding, and poking to make sure that only the best went into her basket. A wave of her hand dismissed the angriest clerk and, although she spoke perfect English, a wave of Hungarian expletives sent them away. She was spending her money and buying health for her family and only the best would do. How many of us were lucky enough to learn about food that way!

If you don't have fruit trees planted in your garden or acres of vegetables outside your window, you must buy your food. Unripe apples are full of starch instead of fruit sugar, oranges are picked green and have color added, bananas are sold green (maybe they'll ripen and maybe they won't). Here are tips on how to spot the best on the shelf, but you still have to protect yourself against the possible fact that some spray may still be on the peel. Wash it well.

Apples

For eating: buy Delicious, McIntosh, Stayman, Jonathan or Winesap. For pies or applesauce, you will want a slightly tart taste. Use Gravenstein, Grimes, Jonathan or Newton. For baking: Rome Beauty, Northern Spy, Winesap, York Imperial. Look for firm, crisp, brightly-colored apples. They should not yield to slight pressure or look at all shriveled. If their stems appear to have been painted, put them back.

Apricots

Look for a uniform, golden-orange color. They should be plump and look as if they're full of juice, and yield to slight pressure. Over-mature fruit is dull-looking, soft or mushy. Immature fruit is very firm and pale yellow or green in color.

Avocados

Turn color as they ripen. Some turn purple-black, others brown or maroon. The texture can be rough or smooth. Look for: slightly soft avocados which yield to gentle pressure on the skin. Avoid avocados with dark, sunken spots in irregular patches or cracked or broken surfaces which are signs of decay. If you use only half of an avocado, leave the pit in and sprinkle lemon juice on it to help prevent browning.

Bananas

Should be firm, bright in appearance and free from bruises or other injuries. The skin color is the indication of ripeness. Look for the skin to be yellow and flecked with brown. That is when the starch in the fruit has been converted to digestible fruit sugar. Never buy a banana with green tips or without yellow color unless you're willing to take a chance on it's ripening. Avoid discolored skins, bruised fruit, a dull, grayish appearance (this usually is a result of frost), or any signs of decay.

Cherries

Wash cherries more than once and with soap and water. Sprays tend to stick to them. Look for the darkest color in sweet cherries. Bing, Black Tartian, Schmidt, Chapman and Republican varieties have colors that range from deep maroon to black. Look for bright, glossy, plump-looking surfaces and fresh-looking stems. Watch out for shriveled, dried stems and a dull appearance, Soft, leaking flesh and brown discoloration is a sign of decay.

Cranberries

Look for plump, firm, berries with lustrous color. They should bounce. Throw away soft, spongy, leaky berries, which can change the flavor and spoil the whole batch.

Grapefruit

They should be heavier than they look. Thin skins mean more juice. Wrinkled skin usually indicates a lot of pulp and little juice. If the peel breaks easily with a little finger pressure or there is a loss of color, put it back. They are signs of decay. Skin defects, scars, etc., usually do not affect the eating quality. Try to buy a well-shaped fruit. If a grapefruit is pointed at the stem end, don't buy it.

Grapes

Thompson seedless: an early green variety. Tokay and Cardinal: early bright reds. Emperor: late deep red.

Concord: blue-black.

Look for well-colored plump fruit with a firm grip on the stem. They shouldn't fall off into your hand. White or green grapes are at their best when they have a slight yellow or amber cast. Red varieties have the best taste when solid color shows throughout. Do not buy wrinkled or soft grapes or those with bleached areas near the stem, or if the fruit is leaking.

Lemons

Look for a rich, yellow natural color with a slightly glossy smooth skin. The fruits should be firm and heavy for their size. Pale or greenish color means they were picked before ripening. Coarse or rough skin indicates a lot of pulp and little juice. Don't buy lemons with punctures, shriveled skin, soft spots, or if they have hardened.

Limes

You want glossy skin and a heavy weight. You don't want dull, dry skin, brown mottling or soft spots—put them back.

Cantaloupe

You can't do much to hurt one of these beauties. Their thick skin is a protection against sprays, you don't have to cook them and they ripen off the vine. They sound ideal and they are. However, there are still things to look for. The color should be yellow-buff or yellow-gray. The veining should be thick, coarse and cork-like. The blossom end should yield to slight pressure and it should have a pleasant odor. If you buy a firm one not quite ready to eat, leave it at room temperature for a few days, then refrigerate for a few hours. Watch for too soft a feel or too yellow a color.

Casaba
Look for gold-yellow rind color and a slight softening at the blossom end. There is no aroma, so don't bother smelling them. Watch for dark, sunken spots. That's decay.

Crenshaw
Look for deep golden-yellow rind with small areas of lighter yellow. The blossom end should yield to moderate thumb pressure. There will be a pleasant aroma. Watch for slightly sunken watersoaked areas on the rind.

Honeydew
Buy when they are ripe and ready to eat—*don't* take them home and wait for them to ripen. They should have a soft feel, a slight softening at the blossom end and a faint fruit aroma. Watch for dead-white or green-white color and a hard, smooth feel, large bruised areas or puncture marks.

Nectarines
Rich color and plumpness. A slight softening along the seam. Bright-looking, moderately hard fruit may ripen at room temperature within two or three days. Watch for dull color, slightly shriveled fruit, soft or overripe or punctured skin.

Oranges
Washington Navel and Valencia should have a thick orange skin color. Temple is excellent for juice and flavor. Look for firm, heavy oranges with bright-looking smooth skin. They should not be green or appear to have been dyed. The acid content in oranges that are picked unripe is too high for pleasant eating. Watch for

light-weight rough- or thick-skinned oranges which lack juice. Dull, dry skin or spongy texture means age and deterioration. Avoid any soft spots, discoloration or splitting around the stem end.

Papaya

Look for a firm, yellowish skin with a tiny yellow ring around the stem. It should smell sweet and give slightly to a light thumb pressure. If it has a heavy odor or the skin caves in at the touch, it is overripe. Papaya is full of enzymes and delightful to eat. Underripe papaya is hard and dark green. That's when it is picked and used for the papain content as a digestant and food tenderizer. This is not what you want to serve yourself or your guests. Put papaya on your shopping list and buy it any time you spot a ripe one.

Mangoes

There are many varieties. Because of that, it's difficult to judge by the color alone. Some start out green and end up spattered with red and gold. That's in the summertime. Other times of the year they can stay green. Look for a little give to the skin and no punctures or overly soft spots. The aroma is enticing. If there's no aroma, there's usually no flavor.

Peaches

The freestone peach is the best for eating. The flesh separates readily from the stone while the clingstone is separated with difficulty. Look for fairly firm, or perhaps slightly soft fruit. The color between the red areas should be yellow. Watch for very firm peaches with a green color between the red areas. They won't ripen properly. Look for any pale tan spot, because that will quickly turn brown and decay.

Pears

Bartlett is the most popular but Anjou, Bosc, Winter Nellis and Comice are available from November into May. Look for firm pears. Bartletts should be pale to rich yellow. Anjou and Comice: light to yellow-green. Bosc: green-yellow to brown-yellow. Winter Nellis: medium to light green. Look for pears that have just begun to soften at the tip.

Persimmons

They're always deep orange, and when they seem to be ready to fall apart, they're ready for eating. If they are not soft and mushy, they are not ripe enough. When ripe they are better than a mouthful of honey. If you do buy them when they are a bit hard, let them stand in the sun for the necessary time. Avoid if they have black spots or leaking.

Pineapples

Come from Hawaii, Mexico and Puerto Rico. The thick skins are a natural protection against chemical sprays. Look for lively color, fragrance, leaves that can be pulled out easily from the top. They should be firm and heavy for their size. Some pineapples start green and, when ripe, turn orange and yellow. But the Sugar Loaf remains green even when it's ripe, so find out if the pineapple is a Sugar Loaf or not. Watch for leaky, soft spots which are signs of decay, and dull yellowish-green color and a dried appearance. Put them back.

Raspberries, Boysenberries, Loganberries

All berries are similar in structure, shape, but differ in color and taste. The quality points are very much the same. Look for bright, clean fruits with a uniform, overall color, plump and tender but not over-soft or mushy. Avoid leaky berries. Inspect the container for wet spots or stains. If they're not up to standard, pass them by. There's a lot of other fruit in the marketplace.

Strawberries
Start in January but the best supply is in May and June. Look for full red color and a bright luster. The flesh should be firm and the cap stem should be firmly attached. The berries will be dry and clean. Turn the basket over and peak at the ones inside. Watch for large uncolored areas or those with large seedy areas. Softness or a dull, shrunken appearance is an indication of decay which can spread very rapidly.

If you want to store the berries for a while, take them out of the container they come in, wash, hull and dry them thoroughly, then put them into a glass container and store in the refrigerator.

Watermelons
It's difficult to judge a watermelon unless it is cut open. Look for firm, juicy flesh with a good red color, free from white streaks. The seeds should be dark brown or black. Watch for a pale colored flesh, white streaks, and white seeds, which indicate immaturity.

Remember, there's no way to get nutrition from a juice unless the nutrition is in the fruit, and, if the fruit is not mature, you're being cheated.

It's not only the money—though certainly that's a problem all by itself—it's the intrinsic value of the vitamin, mineral and enzyme content. It's important to spend some time planning a balanced nutritional diet. It's easy to balance a meal as far as protein, carbohydrate, and fats are concerned. Even calories can be computed with ease, using charts. But the nutritional values are hard to compute. Sometimes certain nutrients are missing from the soil, such as in an area in the United States that is poor in selenium content, and food grown on that soil will also be deficient in that important trace mineral. That's why it is so important to pick the best food you can find and get the most from it.

13. You Are Today What You Ate Yesterday

PROTEIN is the basis of life. It is needed to build and maintain the trillions of body cells, tissues, enzymes, and hormones. It helps to manufacture antibodies, supplies fuel for energy, and countless other procedures that contribute to body health and security.

All proteins are not the same though they are manufactured from the same components. They have different functions and work on different parts of the body. Basically there are two types of protein obtainable from foods: complete and incomplete.

Complete proteins supply the proper balance of the eight necessary amino acids we cannot manufacture in our bodies. These are called essential amino acids because we must get them from the foods we eat. Complete proteins are found mostly in foods of animal origin such as meats, poultry, seafood, eggs, milk and cheeses.

An incomplete protein lacks one or more amino acid, and is not used efficiently for tissue building. However, when a food that is lacking a particular amino acid is combined with another food that supplies the missing amino acid, the result is a complete protein. Examples are combinations of rice and beans or rice and cheese, beans, peas and nuts. (Read *Diet for a Small Planet* by Frances Moore Lappé for combination recipes.)

Vegetarians can have a healthy protein intake without

resorting to animal foods, and the body can be strengthened by the use of fruit and/or vegetable juices if you know the amino acid content of these foods.

It's incorrect to think that vegetables and fruits are accessory foods as so many people do. Too many meals are built around animal protein, with vegetables added as an afterthought or for color. You've seen that fruits and vegetables contain vitamins, minerals, enzymes and so on. Now you'll see the amino acid content.

Alanine

Used in the body for skin and adrenal glands.

Vegetable source:	*Fruit source:*	*Nut source:*
Alfalfa	Apple	Almond
Carrot	Apricot	
Celery	Avocado	
Dandelion greens	Grapes	
Lettuce	Olive	
Cucumber	Orange	
Turnip	Strawberry	
Green pepper		
Spinach		
Watercress		

Arginine

Used in the body for muscle contractions, reproductive organs, cartilage production, body cell regeneration.

Vegetable source:	*Fruit source:*	*Nut source:*
Alfalfa		
Carrot		
Beet		

Vegetable source:	Fruit source:	Nut source:
Cucumber		
Celery		
Lettuce		
Leek		
Radish		
Potato		
Parsnip		

Aspartine

Helps retard bone and teeth destruction, useful for lung and respiratory function, heart and blood vessels.

Vegetable source:	Fruit source:	Nut source:
Carrot	Lemon	Almond
Celery	Grapefruit	
Cucumber	Apple	
Parsley	Apricot	
Radish	Pineapple	
Spinach	Watermelon	
Tomato		
Turnip greens		
Watercress		

Cysteine

Necessary for hair growth, red blood cells, tissue resistance to infection, mammary glands.

Vegetable source:	Fruit source:	Nut source:
Alfalfa	Apple	Brazil nut
Carrot	Currants	Hazel nut
Beet	Pineapple	Filbert

Vegetable source:	Fruit source:	Nut source:
Cabbage	Raspberry	
Cauliflower		
Onion		
Garlic		
Kale		
Horseradish		
Brussels sprouts		

Glutamic Acid

Necessary for insulin production, digestive juices, glycogen formation, acid base balance.

Vegetable source:	Fruit source:	Nut source:
String beans	Papaya	
Brussels sprouts		
Carrot		
Cabbage		
Celery		
Beet greens		
Dandelion greens		
Parsley		
Lettuce		
Spinach		

Glycine

Cartilage, muscle fiber, sex hormones.

Vegetable source:	Fruit source:	Nut source:
Carrot	Fig	Almond
Dandelion greens	Orange	
Turnip	Huckleberry	

Vegetable source:	*Fruit source:*	*Nut source:*
Celery	Raspberry	
Parsley	Pomegranate	
Spinach	Watermelon	
Alfalfa		
Okra		
Garlic		
Potato		

Histidine

Needed for formation of glycogen in the liver, mucus control, blood component.

Vegetable source:	*Fruit source:*	*Nut source:*
Horseradish	Apple	
Radish	Pineapple	
Carrot	Pomegranate	
Beet	Papaya	
Celery		
Cucumber		
Endive		
Leek		
Garlic		
Onion		
Dandelion greens		
Turnip greens		
Alfalfa		
Spinach		
Sorrel		

L-Glutamine
Brain fuel, gastric juices.

Vegetable source:	Fruit source:	Nut source:
Carrot	Grape	
Celery	Huckleberry	
Parsley	Raspberry	
Lettuce	Plum	
Spinach		
Tomato		

Hydroxyproline
Liver and gallbladder, fat emulsifier, red blood cells.

Vegetable source:	Fruit source:	Nut source:
Carrot	Apricot	Almond
Beet	Cherry	Brazil nut
Lettuce	Fig	Coconut
Dandelion greens	Raisin	
Turnip greens	Grapes	
Cucumber	Orange	
	Olive	
	Avocado	
	Pineapple	

Iodogorgoine
All glands (thyroid, lymph, adrenals, etc.).

Vegetable source:	Fruit source:	Nut source:
Dulse	Pineapple	
Kelp		
Sea lettuce		

Vegetable source:	Fruit source:	Nut source:
Carrot		
Celery		
Spinach		
Tomato		
Lettuce		

Isoleucine

Regulation of thymus, spleen, pituitary, hemoglobin, metabolism.

Vegetable source:	Fruit source:	Nut source:
	Papaya	all nuts except pea-
	Avocado	nut, cashew,
	Olive	sunflower

Leucine

Same as Isoleucine

Lysine

Liver and gallbladder, fat metabolism, regulation of pineal gland.

Vegetable source:	Fruit source:	Nut source:
Carrot	Papaya	
Beet	Apple	
Cucumber	Apricot	
Celery	Pear	
Parsley	Grapes	
Spinach		
Dandelion greens		

Vegetable source:	*Fruit source:*	*Nut source:*
Turnip greens		
Alfalfa		
Soybean sprouts		

Methionine

Hemoglobin, tissues, serum, spleen, pancreas, lymph.

Vegetable source:	*Fruit source:*	*Nut source:*
Brussels sprouts	Pineapple	Brazil nut
Cabbage	Apple	Filbert
Cauliflower		
Dock		
Horseradish		
Chive		
Garlic		
Watercress		

Norleucine
Balances other functions

Vegetable source:	*Fruit source:*	*Nut source:*

Must be supplemented or obtained from cheese, eggs or manufactured in the body. As long as there is an adequate supply of all of the other amino acids present, the body will synthesize it.

Phenylalanine
Waste elimination.

Vegetable source:	*Fruit source:*	*Nut source:*
Carrot	Pineapple	

Vegetable source:	Fruit source:	Nut source:
Beet	Apple	
Spinach		
Parsley		
Tomato		

Proline
Regulates fat emulsification.

Vegetable source:	Fruit source:	Nut source:
Carrot	Apricot	Coconut
Beet	Cherry	Almond
Lettuce	Avocado	Brazil nut
Dandelion greens	Fig	
Turnip	Raisin	
Cucumber	Grapes	
	Olive	
	Orange	
	Pineapple	

Serine
Mucous membrane health.

Vegetable source:	Fruit source:	Nut source:
Horseradish	Papaya	
Radish	Apple	
Leek	Pineapple	
Garlic		
Onion		
Carrot		
Beet		
Celery		

Vegetable source:	Fruit source:	Nut source:
Cucumber		
Parsley		
Spinach		
Cabbage		
Alfalfa		

Threonone
Promotes exchange of amino acids to establish balance.

Vegetable source:	Fruit source:	Nut source:
Carrot	Papaya	
Alfalfa		
Green leafy vegetables		

Tryptophane
Generation of cells and tissues, gastric and pancreatic juices, optic system.

Vegetable source:	Fruit source:	Nut source:
Carrot		
Beet		
Celery		
Endive		
Dandelion greens		
Fennel		
Snap beans		
Brussels sprouts		
Chive		
Spinach		
Alfalfa		

Tyrosine

Red blood cells, white blood cells, adrenals, pituitary, thyroid and hair growth.

Vegetable source:	Fruit source:	Nut source:
Alfalfa	Strawberry	Almond
Carrot	Apricot	
Beet	Cherry	
Cucumber	Apple	
Lettuce	Watermelon	
Dandelion greens	Fig	
Parsnip		
Asparagus		
Leek		
Parsley		
Green pepper		
Spinach		
Watercress		

Valine

Glandular functions.

Vegetable source:	Fruit source:	Nut source:
Carrot	Apple	Almond
Turnip	Pomegranate	
Dandelion greens		
Lettuce		
Parsnip		
Squash		
Celery		
Beet		
Parsley		
Okra		
Tomato		

Body Needs of Amino Acids from Outside Sources

Arginine	Methionine
Histidine	Tryptophane
Isoleucine	Phenylalanine
Leucine	Threonine
Lysine	Valine

As you glance over the sources of supply you notice that there are no strangers. All the foods are familiar to you. At one time or other most of them were used as medicines. People versed in tribal lore would gather them and use them when a particular set of symptoms was observed, much the same as certain herbs are used today. How much smarter it is to use them before any symptoms are observed, and how much easier on the system than most chemical medicines! The purpose of this book is to have you think: *prevention*. What diet causes, diet corrects, and you'll never know what you avoided by a correct diet.

Again, it's not necessary to be fanatic about this or any other system. If you observe the rules of healthful eating most of the time, you're ahead of the game.

14. *The Easiest Diet You Ever Tried*

:::

WHAT'S the biggest problem with a diet? Certainly not starting it—that's easy. It's staying on it that's hard.

Do you know the reason it's so hard?

Diets are boring—and somebody else is telling you what to do. It's bad enough to turn the other cheek to the boss, the Internal Revenue Department, the guys who mark up the prices just before you get to the check-out counter, even the kids . . . but when someone else tells you what you can and cannot eat, that's too much.

So listen to me. By the time you get to this chapter you've seen that vegetables and fruits, either whole or in juice form, can supply all the nutrients needed for healthy living. Throw in a couple of nuts and you're home free. If you had to live a vegetarian life, you could. Now hold on to that thought and let's explore a plan to lose weight that puts you in complete control.

Losing weight is a matter of using up more calories than you take in. That's it! No matter what it's called, water diet, Dr. Stillman's diet, Beverly Hills diet, a diet depends on spending more calories than you earn. Older people in particular have trouble with this because some older bodies work less efficiently and there is a gradual decrease in energy production. The caloric needs lessen but the need for vitamins, minerals and other nutrients increases. Older people, in fact, all people, should take vitamins when they go on a diet. It may be okay to miss a meal, but it's not okay to miss your nutrients.

You should adjust your weight by means of a dietary schedule that will cause a weight loss of no more than two pounds a week. That's enough. At the end of three months your scale will show a total loss of twenty-four pounds—and that weight will stay off.

> Fat is figured at 3,500 calories per pound.
> That means you have to spend 7,000 calories to lose two pounds.
> That means you have to eat 7,000 less calories a week.
> Or, 1,000 less calories a day.
> So far, so good!

Now we have to figure how much you need in calories to stay at the weight you are. Forget the average weight charts because nobody is average.

Most adults require 15 calories per pound of body weight to keep their weight constant. Let's calculate based on the case of a woman who weighs in at one hundred forty pounds:

> To stay at one hundred forty pounds she must eat one hundred forty times fifteen equals 2,100 calories a day.
> She would like to lose twenty pounds.
> Since each pound of body fat contains 3,500 calories she must lose 3,500 calories times twenty pounds equals 70,000 calories.

In order to get to the desired weight, our lady must

spend her 70,000 calories. A monumental task? Not at all.

At the rate of two pounds a week (7,000 calories), after ten weeks (70,000 calories total) she will have attained her goal.

Since her present diet of 2,100 calories a day tends to keep her weight constant, she'll have to take in 1,000 less calories a day for ten weeks.

That means ten weeks, only seventy days, eating 1100 calories a day. At the end of ten weeks and when she is at her new, slim, beautiful best, she'll have to recalculate how to eat to keep herself slim. That's done the same way:

> She now weighs one hundred twenty pounds
> One hundred twenty pounds times fifteen equals
> 1800 calories a day.

Isn't it worth a measly seventy days and then you can go back to pizza once in a while!

All of these calculations were necessary to prove that if you reduce your present diet by 1,000 calories a day, then drop an additional one hundred fifty calories after each ten pound weight loss, you'll end up where you want to be on the scale.

> Now what has all of this got to do with vegetables?
> You agree that you could live on vegetables and fruit if you had to!
> Well, you don't have to.
> But they will make up a large part of your next seventy days.
> You don't know how filling 1100 calories can be.
> You're spoiled because one slice of pizza is 540 calories.

A hamburger with all of the trimmings is over 600 calories.

And we haven't touched cake, ice cream, doughnuts, Danish pastry, white bread, candy, soda, milkshakes, malteds, potato chips, french fried potatoes, hot dogs in a bun, burritos . . .

That's where a food-choice chart comes in. You will be able to pick and choose your own menu. Each group supplies a certain number of calories. By picking the foods you want to eat in the quantities that add up to your calorie reduction plan, you'll end up twenty pounds lighter.

FOOD-CHOICE

Group "A" 30 calories per ½ cup	Asparagus	Eggplant
	Green beans	Lettuce
	Broccoli	Mushrooms
	Cabbage	Green pepper
	Cauliflower	Spinach
	Celery	Tomato
	Cucumber	Zucchini

Group "B" 40 calories per ½ cup	Artichokes	Turnips
	Bean sprouts	Brussels sprouts
	Beets	Peas
	Carrots	Squash
	Lima beans	Baked potato
	Rutabagas	

Group "C" 44 calories per ½ cup	Apple	Cantaloupe
	Blackberries	Cherries
	Blueberries	Honeydew melon
	Orange	Huckleberries

Plums	Strawberries
Watermelon	

Group "D"
72 calories
per serving

Wholegrain bread (one slice)
Cooked wholegrain cereal (½ cup)

Group "E"
120 calories
per serving size
of 2 ounces

Beef	Liver
Lamb	Fish
Chicken	Natural cheese
Eggs (two)	Cottage cheese
Turkey	

Group "F"
90 calories per
serving

Avocado (½)
Butter (2 tsp.)
Salad dressing (2 tbsp.)
Whole milk (½ cup)
Skim milk (1 cup)
Unflavored yogurt (½ cup)

Group "G"
155 calories
per serving

Spaghetti (1 cup)
Macaroni (1 cup)
Rice (½ cup)

By choosing your menu from these groups you can
diet on foods you like and still eat only 1100 calories.

For example:

You can plan on 3 servings from group E	360 calories
1 serving from group G	155 calories
2 servings from group D	144 calories
2 servings from group C	88 calories

10 assorted from groups A & B 350 calories
Total   1097calories

Here's the way it looks as a menu:

Breakfast:

Two eggs
One slice of wholegrain bread
Tea with lemon (no sugar)

Lunch:

Vegetable salad (one ½ cup of each)
carrots, peas, bean sprouts, beets,
baked potato.
Dressing of apple cider vinegar and
a dash of lemon
Tea (no sugar)

Snack:

Fresh apple

Dinner:

4 ounces of broiled beef or broiled
fish
1 cup of spaghetti
1 slice wholegrain bread
1½ cups of asparagus
1½ cups of turnips
Salad of cucumber, lettuce and
tomato (one ½ cup of each)
Tea (no sugar)

Snack:

Choice of fruit or ½ cup of milk

That's a lot of food to consume in one day. You will not be hungry as soon as your body adjusts to the new, healthful way of eating. In fact, you'll have more energy, not less.

If, at the end of your program, you decide to stay on the Food-Choice diet you won't be sorry. It is a nutritious plan that you can thrive on for the rest of your life.

Index

Acerola, 116
Acne, 84, 88
Addison's disease, 88–89
Additives, 116
Adenoids, 89
Agar-agar, 116
Alanine, 149
Alfalfa, 27
Allergy, 89
Aluminum, 116–117
Anemia, 21
  cabbage and, 35
  comfrey and, 41
  copper and, 83
  fennel and, 46
  folic acid and, 80
  iron and, 83
  juice formula for, 89–90
  nettle and, 52
  vitamin B6 and, 78–79
  vitamin C and, 81
Antibiotic therapy, 90
Appetite
  carrots and, 37
  chervil and, 40
  currants and, 43
  folic acid and, 80
  gooseberries and, 47
  phosphorus and, 83–84
  sodium and, 84
  vitamin A and, 77
  vitamin B1 and, 77
  vitamin B3 and, 78
  vitamin B12 and, 79
  vitamin C and, 81

Apple, 28, 132–133, 140
Apple swinger, 136
Apricot, 29, 140
Arginine, 149–150
Arrowroot starch, 117
Arteries, 83, 90–91
Arteriosclerosis, 84
Arthritis
  anti-arthritic tea, 43
  celery and, 39
  cherries and, 38
  currants and, 43
  juice formula for, 91
  parsnip and, 58
  vitamin B6 and, 78–79
Artificial flavor and color,
  12, 117
Asparagus, 30
Aspartine, 150
Asthma
  endive and, 45
  juice formula for, 91–92
Avocado, 31, 141

Bacteria, 5, 72
Baking powder, 117
Baking soda, 117
Banana, 31–32, 140–141
Banana flip, 133
Barley, 117–118
Beans (green), 32–33
Beets (red), 33
Beri-beri, 77
Beta-carotene, 14–16,
  28–29, 31, 55

BHA, 117
BHT, 117
Biliousness, 92
Bioflavonoid, 118
Biotin, 80
Blackstrap molasses, 118
Blenders, 70
Boysenberries, 145–146
Breakfast on the run, 137
Brewer's yeast, 9, 118
Bromine, 47, 55, 66–67
Bronchitis
    juice formula for, 93
    peaches and, 59
    pineapple and, 61
Brussels sprouts, 34
Bulgur (bulghar), 118–119
Buttermilk, 119

Cabbage, 34–36
Caffeine, 119
Calcium, 27, 29, 32, 35,
    37, 39, 42–44, 46–47,
    49, 51, 55, 57, 60–61,
    65–67, 81–82
Calorie weight-loss,
    160–166
Canker sores, 78
Cantaloupe, 142
Cantaloupe milk shake,
    133
Carob, 119
Carotene. See Beta-carotene
Carrots, 16, 21, 36–37,
    130, 132–133
Carrot-apple drink, 132
Casaba, 143
Cataracts, 78
Catarrh, 93–94
Celebration drink, 134
Celery, 38–39
Cellulose, 119

Chard, 39–40
Cheese, 119–120
Cherries, 38, 141
Chervil, 40
Chlorine, 43, 58, 60
Chocolate, 120
Cholesterol, 21, 78, 80
Choline, 79
Chromium, 85
Circulation, 94
Citric acid, 49–50, 61
Cobalt, 32, 51
Cocoa, 120
Coconut oil, 120
Coffee, 120
Cold cuts, 120
Colds
    juice formula for, 94
    lemons and, 50
    vitamin P and, 81
Colic, 94
Colitis, 95
Comfrey, 41
Constipation
    copper and, 83
    figs and, 47
    grapes and, 48
    inositol and, 80
    juice formula for, 95
    PABA and, 80
    potassium and, 84
    spinach and, 65
    vitamin D and, 81
Copper, 32, 35, 37, 39,
    51, 55, 57, 60, 65, 68,
    82–83
Corn oil, 124
Corn syrup, 120
Cornell flour formula, 120
Cramps
    calcium and, 82
    parsley and, 57

Cranberry, 130–132, 141
Cranberry-grapefruit mix, 130–131
Crenshaw, 143
Cucumber, 41–42
Currants, 42–43
    black currant syrup, recipe for, 43
Cysteine, 150–151

Dandelion, 44
Depression, 78, 80
Dermatitis, 95–96
Diabetes
    brussels sprouts and, 34
    chromium and, 85
    juice formula for, 96
    strawberries and, 66
Diarrhea, 78, 82, 96–97
Diets, 160–166
Digestion, 4–5
    apple and, 28
    chervil and, 40
    currants and, 43
    fennel and, 46
    folic acid and, 80
    glutamic acid and, 151
    gooseberries and, 47
    grapefruit and, 49
    lemons and, 50
    PABA and, 81
    papaya and, 55
    persimmons and, 60
    sauerkraut and, 36
    vitamin A and, 77
    vitamin B1 and, 77
    vitamin B2 and, 78
    vitamin B6 and, 78
Diuresis
    asparagus and, 30
    carrots and, 37
    celery and, 38

chard and, 40
chervil and, 40
cucumbers and, 42
currants and, 43
gooseberries and, 47
grapefruit and, 49
grapes and, 48
nettle and, 52
parsnip and, 58
Dolomite, 121
Dulse, 121
Dysentery, 97
Dyspepsia
    grapes and, 48

Eczema
    biotin and, 80
    cabbage and, 35
    inositol and, 80
    juice formula for, 97
Emphysema, 97–98
Emulsin, 43
Endive, 45
Enuresis, 98
Enzymes, 4–9, 11
    chart of, 85–86
    destruction of, 6–8, 12–13
    how to obtain, 8–9
    intestinal, 5–6
    salivary, 4
    stomach, 4
    types of, 6
Eyes
    carrots and, 37
    chervil and, 40
    endive and, 45
    fennel and, 46
    inositol and, 80
    juice formula for, 98–99
    parsley and, 57
    tryptophane and, 157
    vitamin A and, 77
    vitamin B2 and, 78

Fasting
  juice-fasting technique,
    48–49, 112–115
Fatigue, 77–78, 81, 84–85,
    99
Fennel, 45–46
Fever, 99
Figs, 46–47
Flatulence, 5
  fennel and, 46
Flours, 121
Folic acid, 28, 44, 62, 65,
    68, 80
Food and Drug
    Administration, 17,
    19, 21
Food labels, 116–128
Food processors, 72
Fools' gold, 134
Fractures, 99–100
Frozen concentrate, 19
Fruit
  how to pick, 139–147
  nutrients in, 17–18
  See also individual
    names of fruits

Gallbladder
  chervil and the, 40
  endive and the, 45
  hydroxyproline and the,
    153
  lysine and the, 154–155
Gallstones
  celery and, 38
  choline and, 79
  juice formula for, 100
Gastritis
  peaches and, 59
  potatoes and, 62
Glutamic acid, 151
Glycine, 151–152

Goiter, 83, 100–101
Gooseberry, 47
Gout
  beans (green) and, 32
  cherries and, 38
  juice formula for, 101
  potatoes and, 62
  strawberries and, 65–66
  watercress and, 69
Grape, 48, 141–142
Grapefruit, 49, 130–132, 141

Hair growth
  biotin and, 80
  cucumbers and, 42
  cysteine and, 150–151
  inositol and, 80
  iodine and, 83
  juice formula for, 102
  lettuce and, 51
  parsnip and, 58
  sulphur and, 84
  tyrosine and, 158
  vitamin B2 and, 78
  vitamin B5 and, 78
  vitamin B6 and, 78–79
  vitamin E and, 82
  watercress and, 68
Halitosis, 78
Hay fever
  endive and, 45
  juice formula for, 102
Headaches, 78, 81, 102–103
Heart, 77, 80–84, 150
Hemorrhoids
  chard and, 40
  juice formula for,
    101–102
  nettle and, 52
  turnips and, 68
High blood pressure, 79
Histidine, 152

Honey, 9, 11, 39, 121–122, 133–138
Honeydew, 143
Honey/fruit punch, 133
Hot cider punch, 136
Hot dogs, 122
Hydraulic press, 72
  Norwalk Hydraulic press, 73–74
Hydrochloric acid, 5
Hydrogenated, 122
Hydroxyproline, 153
Hypoglycemia, 78, 85

Indigestion, 103
Influenza, 104
Inositol, 80
Insect bites
  lemons and, 50
Insomnia, 78, 80–82
Iodine, 35, 39, 51, 57, 60–61, 63, 65–66, 68, 83
Iodogorgoine, 153–154
Irish moss, 122
Iron, 21, 27, 29–30, 35, 37, 39, 40, 44, 46–47, 51, 55, 57, 61, 65–68, 77, 83
Isoleucine, 154

Juice extractor, 8, 14
  Acme Juicerator, 75
  the Braun Juicer, 73
  the Champion Juicer, 73
  how to buy, 70–75
  the Phoenix Juicer, 74
  Vitamix, 74–75
Juices
  benefits of, 10–15, 24–25

formulas of, 88–111, 129–138
nutrients in, 16–25
See also individual names of juices; Diets

Kasha, 122
Kefir, 8, 122
Kelp, 9, 51, 68, 122
Kidney ailments
  apple and, 28
  bananas and, 32
  bladder troubles, juice formula for, 92–93
  choline and, 79
  inositol and, 80
  juice formula for, 104
  pineapples and, 61
  radishes and, 63
  vitamin B5 and, 78

Laryngitis, 104–105
Laxative
  bananas as a, 32
  celery as a, 38
  chard as a, 40
  currants as a, 43
  prunes as a, 60
  rhubarb as a, 64
  strawberries as a, 65
Lecithin, 122–123
Legumes, 123
Lemons, 49–50, 142
Lettuce, 50–52
Leucine, 154
Limes, 142
Lipids, 29, 62
Liver
  chervil and the, 40
  choline and the, 79
  endive and the, 45
  histidine and, 152

hydroxyproline and, 153
inositol and the, 80
juice formula for, 105
lysine and the, 154–155
strawberries and the, 66
Loganberries, 145–146
Low blood pressure,
     105–106
Lungs
  aspartine and the, 150
  cancer of, 14
  parsnips and the, 58
  vitamin E and the, 82
  watercress and the, 69
Lysine, 154–155

Magnesium, 27, 29, 37, 39,
     43–44, 51, 55, 57,
     60–61, 63, 65–68, 83
Malic acid, 28, 43, 48, 61
Malt, 123
Manganese, 30, 37, 39, 42,
     47, 55, 57, 60–61, 65
Mangoes, 144
Maple sugar, 123
Melon, 52–53
Menopause, 106–107
Menstruation
  disturbances, 79
  juice formulas for, 106
Methionine, 155
Milk of the lion, 138
Mineral oil, 124
Minerals, 11, 13
  chart of, 86–87
  See also individual
     names of minerals
Miscarriage, 82
MSG, 123
Mucous membrane, 107,
     152, 156–157
Muesli, 8

Mulberry, 53–54
Mulled apple juice, 131
Myopia, 81
Mystery drink, 131

Nectarines, 143
Nervous disorders
  calcium and, 82
  celery and, 39
  choline and, 79
  juice formula for,
     107–108
  PABA and, 81
  phosphorus and, 84
  potassium and, 84
  strawberries and, 66
  vitamin B1 and, 77
  vitamin B3 and, 78
  vitamin D and, 81
Nettle, 52
Niacin, 28, 78
Nitrilosides, 29
Non-dairy milk product,
     123
Norleucine, 155

Obesity, 83
Oils, 124–125
Olive oil, 124
Orange, 54–55, 143–144
  juice of, 17, 19
  Nectar drink, 132
Organ meats, 125
Oxalic acid, 1–2, 64–65

PABA, 80–81
Papain, 55
Papaya, 9, 55–56, 144
Parsley, 56–58
Parsnip, 58
Pasteurization
  of orange juice, 19

Peaches, 59, 144
Peanut butter, 125–126
Peanut oil, 124
Pear cooler, 135
Pears, 59, 145
Pectin, 21–22, 28, 43, 49
Pepsin, 5, 60
Persimmons, 59, 145
Phenylalanine, 155–156
Phosphorus, 16, 28–29, 32–33, 35, 37, 39, 42–43, 46–47, 49, 51, 55, 57–58, 60–61, 65–67, 83–84
Pick-me-up, 131
Pineapple, 60–61, 130, 145
Pineapple-carrot surprise, 130
Plantains, 59
Plums, 59–60
Poisons
  oxalic acid, 1
  wild parsnips, 58
Polyunsaturates, 126
Potassium, 16–17, 27–30, 33, 37, 39, 42–44, 46–47, 51, 55, 57–58, 60–61, 63, 65–67, 84
Potato, 61–62
Preservatives
  in canned foods, 12
Proline, 156
Prostate trouble, 108
Protein, 29, 31, 35, 41, 43, 55–56, 62, 148–159
Pumpkin seeds, 126

Radish, 63
Raspberries, 145–146
Raw juice. *See* Juices
Raw vegetables. *See* Vegetables

Recipes. *See* Juices, formulas for
Respiratory ills
  alfalfa and, 27–28
  aspartine and, 150
  vitamin A and, 77
  vitamin B3 and, 78
Rheumatism
  beans (green) and, 32
  cucumbers and, 42
  juice formula for, 108–109
  lemons and, 50
Rhubarb, 64
Rice, 126
Rickets, 81
Ricotta, 126
Rutin, 30

Safflower oil, 124
Salad dressings, 126–127
Salt
  balanced by potassium, 17
  -free diet, 127
  in canned foods, 12
Sauerkraut, 8, 36
Schizophrenia, 79
Scurvy, 81
Selenium, 84, 147
Serine, 156–157
Sesame oil, 125
Sex
  celery and, 39
  glycine and, 151–152
  juice formula for, 109
  vitamin B3 and, 78
Sexy vegetable juice, 136
Silicon, 27, 42, 58, 66
Sinus problems
  alfalfa and, 27–28
  juice formula for, 109
  vitamin A and, 77

Skin
  alanine and the, 149
  avocado and the, 31
  biotin and the, 80
  grapes and the, 48
  iron and the, 83
  juice formula for, 109–110
  lemons and the, 50
  potassium and the, 84
  strawberries and the, 66
  vitamin A and the, 77
  vitamin B2 and the, 78
  vitamin B3 and the, 78
  vitamin B5 and the, 78
Sodium, 27, 29, 37, 39,
    42–44, 55, 60, 63,
    65–66, 84
Soft drinks, 127
Sorghum, 127
South Sea delight, 135
Soy oil, 125
Soy sauce, 127
Spinach, 64–65
Sterility
  vitamin A and, 77
  vitamin E and, 82
  zinc and, 85
Sterilization
  in canning process, 12
Strawberry, 65–66, 129, 146
Strawberry shaky, 129
Sugar
  brown sugar, 11
  digestion of, 12
  in grapefruit, 49
  in melons, 53
  refined, 10–11
  sugar beet, 11
  sugar cane, 11
Sulfur, 29, 33, 35, 37, 42,
    46, 57–58, 60–61,
    65–66, 68, 84

Summer freshener, 134
Summer pick-up, 132
Sunflower oil, 125
Sweeteners, natural, 127

Tahini, 127
Tannic acid, 28, 48, 54
Tapioca, 127
Teeth
  aspartine and, 150
  carrots and, 37
  juice formula for, 93
  turnips and, 67
  vitamin C and, 81
  vitamin D and, 81
Thick shake, 137
Thirst quencher, 135
Threonone, 157
Tomato, 66–67, 129
Tryptophane, 157
Turnip, 67–68
Tyrosine, 158

Ulcers, 21
  bananas and, 32
  cabbage and, 35
  carrots and, 37
  choline and, 79
  comfrey and, 41
  juice formula for, 108
  potatoes and, 62
  vitamin B1 and, 77
  vitamin C and, 81
Urinary tract infections
  chard and, 40
  parsley and, 57
  vitamin A and, 77

Valine, 158
Vanilla, 128
Varicosity, 110
Vegetable seasoning, 128

Vegetables
  cooking of, 13–14
  nutrients in, 20–21
  raw, 23–25
  See also individual names
    of vegetables
Vinegar, 128
Vitamin gold mine, 137
Vitamins, 4, 11
  A, 14, 27, 29–33, 35,
    37, 39–40, 42, 44–47,
    49, 51, 53–54, 56,
    60–61, 65–68, 77
  B, 13, 27–30, 32–33, 35,
    37, 39, 41–42, 44,
    46–47, 51, 53, 55, 57,
    60–61, 63, 65–68, 77–79
  C, 13, 19, 21, 27–30,
    32–34, 37, 39–40,
    42–44, 46–47, 49, 51,
    53–56, 60–61, 63,
    65–68, 81
  chart for, 85–86
  D, 27, 31, 37, 51, 61,
    63, 81
  E, 27, 31–32, 37, 51,
    63, 66, 82
  K, 27, 37, 66–67, 82
  P, 49, 55, 60, 63, 81
  supplemental, 17
  U, 27, 36

Waist-watcher, 138
Watercress, 68–69
Watermelon, 146–147
Watermelon-ade, 132
Water retention, 110
Weight loss, 160–165
Wheat germ oil, 125
Whey, 128
Wine press, 72
Wounds
  comfrey and, 41
  juice formula for, 110–111

Yogurt, 8, 128
Yogurt-tomato mix, 129–130

Zinc, 51, 55, 65, 85

The Best in Health Books by
LINDA CLARK, BEATRICE TRUM HUNTER and CARLSON WADE

By Linda Clark

☐ **Know Your Nutrition** — $4.95
☐ **Face Improvement Through Nutrition** — $2.25
☐ **Be Slim and Healthy** — $1.50
☐ **Go-Caution-Stop Carbohydrate Computer** — $1.95
☐ **The Best of Linda Clark** — $4.50
☐ **How to Improve Your Health** — $4.95

By Beatrice Trum Hunter

☐ **Whole Grain Baking Sampler**
   ☐ Cloth $6.95   ☐ Paperback $2.95
☐ **Additives Book** — $2.25
☐ **Fermented Foods and Beverages** — $1.25
☐ **Yogurt, Kefir & Other Milk Cultures** — $1.75
☐ **Wheat, Millet and Other Grains** — $1.45
☐ **High Power Foods** — $1.45

By Carlson Wade

☐ **Arthritis and Nutrition** — $1.95
☐ **Bee Pollen** — $2.50
☐ **Lecithin** — $2.25
☐ **Fats, Oils and Cholesterol** — $1.50
☐ **Vitamins and Other Supplements** — $1.50
☐ **Hypertension (High Blood Pressure) and Your Diet** — $1.95

Buy them at your local health or book store or use this coupon.

Keats Publishing, Inc. (P.O. Box 876), New Canaan, Conn. 06840
Please send me the books I have checked above. I am enclosing
$_____ (add $1.00 to cover postage and handling). Send check
or money order — no cash or C.O.D.'s please.

Mr/Mrs/Miss _____

Address_____

City_____State_____Zip_____
(Allow three weeks for delivery)

COOKBOOKS ON NATURAL HEALTH
... To Help You Eat Better for Less!

☐ **ADD A FEW SPROUTS** (Martha H. Oliver)   **$1.95**

☐ **WHOLE GRAIN BAKING SAMPLER**
    (Beatrice Trum Hunter)   **$2.95**

☐ **MRS. APPLEYARD'S KITCHEN** (L.A. Kent)   **$3.95**

☐ **MRS. APPLEYARD'S SUMMER KITCHEN**
    (L.A. Kent & E.K. Gay)   **$3.95**

☐ **MRS. APPLEYARD'S WINTER KITCHEN**
    (L.A. Kent & E.K. Gay)   **$3.95**

☐ **BETTER FOODS FOR BETTER BABIES**
    (Gena Larson)   **$2.25**

☐ **GOOD FOODS THAT GO TOGETHER**
    (Esther L. Smith)   **$3.95**

☐ **MEALS AND MENUS FOR ALL SEASONS**
    (Agnes Toms)   **$1.25**

☐ **NATURAL FOODS BLENDER COOKBOOK**
    (Frieda Nusz)   **$1.95**

☐ **BONNIE FISHER'S WAY WITH HERBS**   **$2.95**

☐ **GOOD FOOD, GLUTEN FREE** (Hilda Cherry Hills)   **$4.50**

☐ **LOAVES AND FISHES**
    (Malvina Kinard & Janet Crisler)   **$4.95**

☐ **MENNONITE COMMUNITY COOKBOOK**
    (Mary Emma Showalter)   **$1.75**

☐ **EAT THE WEEDS** (Ben Charles Harris)   **$1.50**

Buy them at your local health or book store or use this coupon.

Keats Publishing, Inc. (P.O. Box 876), New Canaan, Conn. 06840   75-G
Please send me the books I have checked above. I am enclosing
$_____(add $1.00 to cover postage and handling). Send check
or money order — no cash or C.O.D.'s please.

Mr/Mrs/Miss_____

Address_____

City_____ State_____ Zip_____
       (Allow three weeks for delivery.)